ADVANCES IN IMAGING TECHNIQUES IN ISCHEMIC HEART DISEASE

Developments in Cardiovascular Medicine

VOLUME 171

ADVANCES IN IMAGING TECHNIQUES IN ISCHEMIC HEART DISEASE

edited by

ERNST E. VAN DER WALL

Department of Cardiology,
University Hospital Leiden,
Leiden, The Netherlands

THOMAS H. MARWICK

Department of Cardiology,
Cleveland Clinic Foundation,
Cleveland, U.S.A.

and

JOHAN H.C. REIBER

Department of Diagnostic Radiology,
University Hospital Leiden,
Leiden, The Netherlands

BYK

SPRINGER-SCIENCE+BUSINESS MEDIA, B.V.

A C.I.P. Catalogue record for this book is available from the Library of Congress.

CIP-DATA ROYAL LIBRARY, THE HAGUE

Advances

ed. : E.E. van der Wall, Th.H. Marwick, J.H.C. Reiber. - Leiden :
Boerhaave Commissie voor Postacademisch Onderwijs in de
Geneeskunde, Rijksuniversiteit Leiden. - (Boerhaave
cursus, ISSN 0929-8940).
Symposium georganiseerd door Departments of Cardiology, and Diagnostic Radiology-
and Nuclear Medicine of the University Hospital Leiden en Cleveland Clinic
International Center, zaterdag 19 augustus 1995. - Met lit. opg.
ISBN 978-94-010-4163-8 ISBN 978-94-011-0365-7 (eBook)
DOI 10.1007/978-94-011-0365-7
Trefw.: hartziekten: beeldverwerkende diagnostiek.

ISBN 978-94-010-4163-8

Printed on acid-free paper

We gratefully acknowledge the financial support of:

Byk Nederland B.V.

Amersham Nederland B.V.
Bristol-Myers Squibb
Philips Medical Systems
Siemens Medical Engineering
Sonotron B.V.

Contents

List of contributors

J. Baan
Department of Cardiology, University Hospital Leiden, P.O. Box 9600, 2300 RC, Leiden, the Netherlands

M.A. Bekedam
Department of Cardiology, University Hospital Leiden, P.O. Box 9600, 2300 RC, Leiden, the Netherlands

C. von Birgelen
Thoraxcenter, University Hospital Rotterdam-Dijkzigt, Dr. Molenwaterplein 40, 3015 GD Rotterdam, the Netherlands

N. Bom
Thoraxcenter, Erasmus University, P.O. Box 1738, 3000 DR, Rotterdam, the Netherlands

A.V.G. Bruschke
Department of Cardiology, University Hospital Leiden, P.O. Box 9600, 2300 RC, Leiden, the Netherlands

J. Doornbos
Department of Diagnostic Radiology and Nuclear Medicine, University Hospital Leiden, P.O. Box 9600, 2300 RC, Leiden, the Netherlands

J.J. Gerbrands
Information Theory group, Delft University of Technology, P.O. Box 5, 2600 AA, Delft, the Netherlands

B. Goedhart
Department of Diagnostic Radiology and Nuclear Medicine, University Hospital Leiden, P.O. Box 9600, 2300 RC, Leiden, the Netherlands

E.J. Gussenhoven
Thoraxcenter, Erasmus University, P.O. Box 1738, 3000 DR, Rotterdam, the Netherlands

J.W. Jukema
Department of Cardiology, University Hospital Leiden, P.O. Box 9600, 2300 RC, Leiden, the Netherlands

G. Koning
Department of Diagnostic Radiology and Nuclear Medicine, University Hospital Leiden, P.O. Box 9600, 2300 RC, Leiden, the Netherlands

C.L. de Korte
Thoraxcenter, Erasmus University, P.O. Box 1738, 3000 DR, Rotterdam, the Netherlands

C.T. Lancée
Thoraxcenter, Erasmus University, P.O. Box 1738, 3000 DR, Rotterdam, the Netherlands

W. Li
Thoraxcenter, Erasmus University, P.O. Box 1738, 3000 DR, Rotterdam, the Netherlands

P.R. Luyten
Philips Medical Systems, MR Clinical Science, P.O. Box 10000, 5680 DA, Best, the Netherlands

Th.H. Marwick
Department of Cardiology, Cleveland Clinic International Center, 9500 Euclid Avenue, Cleveland 44195, U.S.A.

P.M.T. Pattynama
Department of Diagnostic Radiology and Nuclear Medicine, University Hospital Leiden, P.O. Box 9600, 2300 RC, Leiden, the Netherlands

J.H.C. Reiber
Department of Diagnostic Radiology and Nuclear Medicine, University Hospital Leiden, P.O. Box 9600, 2300 RC, Leiden, the Netherlands

A. de Roos
Department of Diagnostic Radiology and Nuclear Medicine, University Hospital Leiden, P.O. Box 9600, 2300 RC, Leiden, the Netherlands

M.J. Schalij
Department of Cardiology, University Hospital Leiden, P.O. Box 9600, 2300 RC, Leiden, the Netherlands

L.R. Schiemanck
Department of Diagnostic Radiology and Nuclear Medicine, University Hospital Leiden, P.O. Box 9600, 2300 RC, Leiden, the Netherlands

A.F.W. van der Steen
Thoraxcenter, Erasmus University, P.O. Box 1738, 3000 DR, Rotterdam, the Netherlands

J. Thomas
Department of Cardiology, Cleveland Clinic International Center, 9500 Euclid Avenue, Cleveland 44195, U.S.A.

E.M. Tuzcu
Department of Cardiology, Cleveland Clinic International Center, 9500 Euclid Avenue, Cleveland 44195, U.S.A.

H.W. Vliegen
Department of Cardiology, University Hospital Leiden, P.O. Box 9600, 2300 RC, Leiden, the Netherlands

E.E. van der Wall
Department of Cardiology, University Hospital Leiden, P.O. Box 9600, 2300 RC, Leiden, the Netherlands

P.M.J. van der Zwet
Department of Diagnostic Radiology and Nuclear Medicine, University Hospital Leiden, P.O. Box 9600, 2300 RC, Leiden, the Netherlands

Preface

In recent years there have been tremendous advances in cardiac imaging techniques covering the complete spectrum from echocardiography, nuclear cardiology, magnetic resonance imaging to contrast angiography. With respect to these noninvasive and invasive cardiac imaging modalities, marked technological developments have allowed the cardiologist to visualize the myocardium in a far more refined manner than conventional imaging was capable of. Echocardiography has extended its domain with intravascular ultrasound, cardiovascular nuclear imaging has added positron emission tomography to its line of research, magnetic resonance imaging has been broadened with magnetic resonance angiography and spectroscopy, and finally contrast angiography has widened its scope with excellent quantitation programs. For all these imaging modalities it is true that the application of dedicated quantitative analytic software packages enables the evaluation of the imaging studies in a more accurate, reliable, and reproducible manner. It goes without saying that these extensions and achievements have resulted in improved diagnostics and subsequently in improved patient care. Particularly in patients with ischemic heart disease, major progress has been made to detect coronary artery disease in an early phase of the disease process, to follow the atherosclerotic changes in the coronary arteries, to establish the functional and metabolic consequences of the luminal obstructions, and to accurately assess the results of interventional therapy. For instance, intravascular ultrasound permits the early detection of coronary artery disease, magnetic resonance angiography can presently be used for screening of disease, nuclear imaging techniques using positron emission tomography may well be applied for evaluation of the functional and metabolic consequences of coronary artery lesions, and quantitative coronary angiography allows the assessment of successful interventional therapy.

Advances in Imaging Techniques in Ischemic Heart Disease is a bibliographical 'image' of a Symposium, held on August 19, 1995, in Leiden. At this Symposium all major advances in cardiac imaging techniques in ischemic heart disease were addressed varying from intravascular ultrasound to positron emission tomography, and from magnetic resonance coronary angiography to quantitative contrast coronary angiography. In addition, major attainments in conventional imaging approaches were discussed such as new tracers for myocardial perfusion imaging, developments in contrast and stress echocardiography, and stress magnetic resonance imaging. Finally, the value of the various cardiac imaging techniques was highlighted in order to emphasize their important role in assessing the effects of interventional therapy such as early reperfusion and lipid lowering drugs. Based on the presentations of all speakers, this book consists of a compilation of manuscripts related to each of these specific topics.

Herewith we like to acknowledge all individuals, societies, and institutions who have had a substantial contribution to our Symposium and therefore to the appearance of *Advances in Imaging Techniques in Ischemic Heart Disease*. First of all, we believe that the Symposium was unique because of three factors; 1) the Symposium was a joint venture between Leiden University Hospital and Cleveland Clinic International Center, 2) the Symposium was an international Boerhaave Course which has by nature a long-standing reputation, and 3) the Symposium included the prestigious Einthoven Lecture, this year presented by René G. Favoloro, Buenos Aires, Argentina. We express our gratitude to all authors and co-authors for making great efforts in preparing their superb up-to-date chapters at short-term. The authors are all excellent investigators in one or more fields of cardiac imaging and they have stimulated progress in cardiac imaging with the aim to improve patient care. We like to acknowledge our sponsors i.e. the Netherlands Society of Cardiology (NVVC), the Interuniversity Cardiology Institute of the Netherlands (ICIN), the Einthoven Foundation, the Cleveland Clinic Foundation (CCF), and Cleveland Clinic International Center (CCIC). We like to thank the Departments of Cardiology (Head Prof.dr. A.V.G. Bruschke), Radiology (Head Prof.dr. A.E. van Voorthuisen) and Nuclear Medicine (Head Prof.dr. E.K.J. Pauwels) of the Leiden University for their support in organizing the Symposium. In part, this book may also be considered as a mark of honour to Prof.dr. A.V.G. Bruschke who at the time of the Symposium has been head of the Department of Cardiology for a period of exactly 10 years as he moved from the St. Antonius Hospital (Nieuwegein, The Netherlands) to Leiden University in August 1985. We are very grateful to Dr. M. Razavi (Cleveland Clinic International Center) who as a Course Director, together with Prof. Bruschke, took the initiative to this joint Symposium and laid the basis for an excellent bilateral program. We are very much indebted to Mrs A.E.H. Zitter and Mr J.J.L. Muller (Boerhaave Committee, Leiden, The Netherlands) who superbly assisted us in organizing the Symposium. We like to acknowledge Mrs N. Dekker (Kluwer Academic Publishers, Dordrecht, The Netherlands) and Mr J. Schoones (Leiden University Medical Library) who, together with Mrs A.E.H. Zitter, put a lot of effort in editing, preparing, and completing *Advances in Imaging Techniques in Ischemic Heart Disease*. Lastly, the appearance of this book would not have been possible without a generous grant from Byk Nederland B.V. (Zwanenburg, The Netherlands).

We hope that this book will assist the cardiologist, the radiologist, the nuclear medicine physician, physicists, basic scientists, and the fellows who are in training for those specialties, in understanding the most recent achievements in cardiac imaging techniques in ischemic heart disease.

The Editors
Ernst E. van der Wall, Thomas H. Marwick, Johan H.C. Reiber

Current status of myocardial perfusion scintigraphy

E.E. van der Wall
Department of Cardiology, University Hospital Leiden, the Netherlands

Summary

Over the last decade, substantial advancements in the field of myocardial perfusion scintigraphy have markedly improved the diagnosis and subsequent evaluation of patients with coronary artery disease (CAD). These improvements have originated from the development of single photon emission computed tomography (SPECT), the addition of several new technetium-99m (^{99m}Tc) based radiopharmaceuticals into clinical practice, and the introduction of pharmacological stress agents. Yet, thallium-201 (^{201}Tl) has kept its role as the predominant tracer for assessment of myocardial viability. In this era of continuing cost containment, myocardial perfusion scintigraphy has emerged as a highly cost effective noninvasive modality for guiding patient management.

Introduction

Over the past 5 years, several myocardial perfusion agents labeled with ^{99m}Tc have become commercially available. One of them, ^{99m}Tc-sestamibi (Cardiolite) has already been in clinical use in several countries around the world [1]. Another agent, ^{99m}Tc-teboroxime (Cardiotec), has been approved for clinical use but has had much less clinical utilization. The newest ^{99m}Tc-labeled perfusion agent that has undergone clinical evaluation is ^{99m}Tc-tetrofosmin (Myoview) [2]. The advent of these compounds occurred 15-20 years after the introduction of myocardial perfusion scintigraphy in 1976 as a clinical tool using ^{201}Tl as a tracer. In the coming years, the new ^{99m}Tc-labeled agents will in all likelihood radically change the ways one performs myocardial perfusion scintigraphy. Because of the constraints imposed by the physical characteristics of ^{201}Tl - such as the low emission energies (68 to 80 keV) resulting in severe photon attenuation, the long half-life (73 hours) limiting the maximal injected dose to only a few millicuries (megabecquerels), and the need to be produced in a cyclotron, ^{201}Tl has

E. E. van der Wall et al. (eds.), Advances in Imaging Techniques in Ischemic Heart Disease 1–16.

been considered a relatively poor perfusion tracer when imaged with single-crystal gamma cameras. Consequently, nuclear medicine physicians and cardiologists have searched for other tracers such as ^{99m}Tc, which is a much more favorable agent for the current generation of gamma cameras (half-life 6 hours, emission energy 140 keV). Now that these tracers have been developed, ^{201}Tl is receiving a second look. The need for this second look emerges from a wealth of data that have definitely established the powerful diagnostic and prognostic value of ^{201}Tl scintigraphy. This value has been enhanced recently by important advances, such as 1) the introduction of SPECT, 2) the potential of ^{201}Tl reinjection to enhance the detection of viable myocardium, and 3) the use of potent coronary vasodilators such as dipyridamole and adenosine, which enhance myocardial ^{201}Tl uptake. The main question is whether all the prognostic indicators, which have been extensively validated with respect to ^{201}Tl scintigraphy, will also apply to the ^{99m}Tc-labeled agents. In this regard one should wait until prognostic data using the ^{99m}Tc agents are forthcoming. Currently, none of the newer agents has been shown to be clearly superior to ^{201}Tl.
This chapter will concentrate on the merits of SPECT imaging, the use of the appropriate imaging protocols -both for ^{201}Tl and ^{99m}Tc-sestamibi-, and the application of pharmacologic stress in myocardial perfusion imaging.

Planar versus SPECT imaging

Planar myocardial perfusion scintigraphy is a time-honored technique for diagnosing patients with CAD and is widely accessible, simple to perform, allows accurate quantitative analysis, and requires less quality control than SPECT [3]. However, with planar imaging there is significant overlap of normally and abnormally perfused myocardium which limits its overall diagnostic accuracy. SPECT, an inherently three-dimensional technique, can overcome many of the limitations of planar imaging and is more accurate for the overall detection and localization of coronary artery stenosis [4].

SPECT quantification

A well-recognized advantage of SPECT is the ability to accurately quantify the global extent of left ventricular hypoperfusion and the percent of myocardial scar and ischemia. Although different software packages are currently available, all are based principally on a circumferential profile technique whereby pixel count activity is determined along radii from the left ventricular endocardium to epicardium over the entire 360 degrees of each stress and redistribution (or rest) short axis slice from cardiac apex to base. The count activity for each radius is normalized to the radius with the highest activity in each of the initial stress and delayed short axis slices. Two-dimensional polar maps of the three-dimensional myocardial radionuclide activity are then computer-generated (bull's eye reconstruction) and statistically compared to a normal patient data bank. Quantification with SPECT has been validated in models of experimental infarction, and also in clinical trials comparing scintigraphic infarct size to enzymatic estimates of myocardial infarction [5]. The unique ability of SPECT to quantify the extent of myocardial scar and ischemia is now recognized to confer important prognostic information.

Reproducibility of SPECT

In large multicenter trials, mean patient data are used to assess the efficacy of different therapeutic regimens, but in clinical practice individual efficacy becomes the critical issue. In order to define what constitutes a real change in myocardial perfusion beyond technique variability, the reproducibilities of both planar and SPECT imaging have recently been investigated [6]. The intra- and interobserver reproducibility of SPECT for quantifying perfusion defects proved to be excellent with correlation coefficients of $r=.99$ and $r=.98$, respectively, ($p<.0001$). Furthermore, the inter-study reproducibility was equally high.

Myocardial imaging with ^{201}Tl

Thallium-201 perfusion imaging has been used with excellent clinical results for almost 20 years. Since 1977 the traditional exercise-delayed imaging protocol has been used in millions of patients. According to the traditional imaging protocol the patient performs symptom-limited exercise on a treadmill or bicycle. At peak exercise 2-3 mCi (75-110 MBq) of ^{201}Tl is injected intravenously. The patient is encouraged to continue to exercise for 1 to 2 more minutes. The patient is then positioned as soon as possible under the gamma camera (within 5-10 minutes after termination of exercise). Delayed redistribution imaging is performed 2-4 hours after injection of ^{201}Tl.

Several new protocols have been recently proposed in ^{201}Tl myocardial perfusion imaging. It has been shown that, with the above-described conventional ^{201}Tl imaging protocol, the reversibility of exercise-induced perfusion defects, and thus myocardial viability, may be underestimated. Depending on the population studied, 40-60% of patients with fixed defects may have viable myocardium in the defect area. The traditional 2-4 hour delay is apparently too short for complete redistribution of ^{201}Tl to

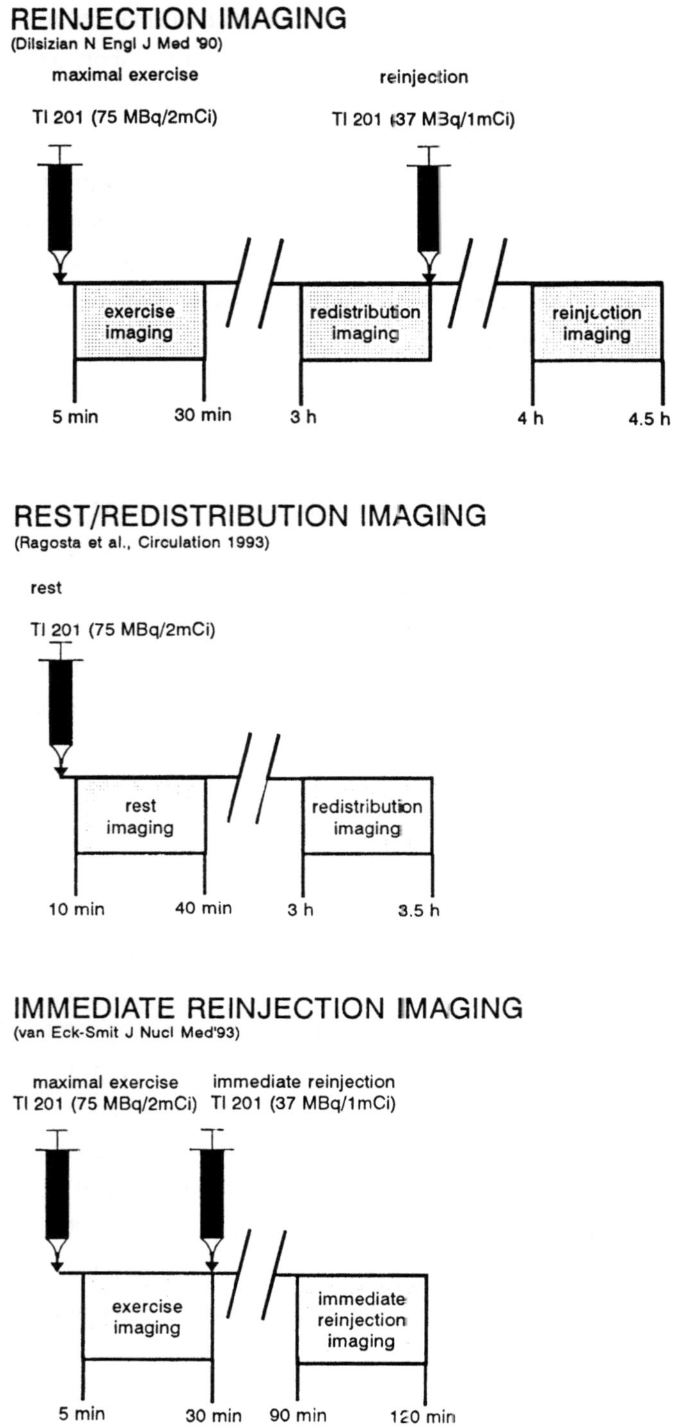

Fig. 1: Currently established protocols for ^{201}Tl myocardial imaging in the detection of perfusion and viability.

occur. To circumvent this limitation a number of alternative protocols have been developed for the combined assessment of perfusion and viability.

A first protocol uses late redistribution imaging to be performed 24 hours after injection of ^{201}Tl in patients with fixed defects on conventional 2-4 hour delayed imaging [7]. This modification requires no additional injection of ^{201}Tl. However, the count density is usually low 24 hours after injection, resulting in suboptimal images. Compared with imaging after a rest reinjection, less defect reversibility is detected [8].

In a subsequent more efficient protocol, for the first time described by Dilzisian et al. in 1990 [9], ^{201}Tl is reinjected at rest as soon as 3-4 hour redistribution imaging is completed (classical reinjection protocol). Imaging is started 30 to 45 minutes after rest reinjection and complete evaluation by ^{201}Tl imaging is achieved in one day. Despite the relatively long imaging procedure of 5-6 hours, the standard stress-redistribution-reinjection protocol has been accepted as a routine procedure in many nuclear medicine laboratories [10].

A newly proposed elegant imaging protocol is the socalled stress-immediate reinjection procedure, initially proposed by Van Eck-Smit et al. in 1993 [11], whereby ^{201}Tl is reinjected at rest as soon as exercise imaging is completed. Delayed rest imaging is performed 1 hour after the rest injection. The total procedure is much shorter (2.5 hours) than the conventional ^{201}Tl imaging protocol or the classical reinjection protocol. In a quantitative comparative analysis of the stress-stress-redistribution-reinjection approach versus the stress-immediate reinjection approach in the same patient, excellent agreement existed for perfusion defect size and defect reversibility [12]. Another variation of this modification involves the administration of 20 mg isosorbide dinitrate orally after exercise before ^{201}Tl reinjection [13].

A next approach consists of a continuous infusion over 4 hours of 1.5 mCi (55 MBq) of ^{201}Tl given after completion of exercise imaging [14]. The total imaging time is similar to that of the conventional imaging protocol. Theoretically, it should be the ideal approach for assessing viability in hibernating myocardium. It is inconvenient, however; the patient is required to stay in the laboratory for the slow infusion of ^{201}Tl. Further clinical validation of this procedure is needed.

A last ^{201}Tl-imaging protocol is the so-called rest-redistribution imaging, first described by Ragosta et al. in 1993 [15]. In contrast to the ^{201}Tl exercise protocols, the rest-4-hour redistribution procedure is mainly reserved for identifying viable tissue in patients with moderate to severe ischemic left ventricular dysfunction and can predict functional recovery after coronary bypass procedures.

Although each of the aforementioned approaches has its own merits, the most practical approach for exercise ^{201}Tl imaging is, in my opinion, to follow the stress-immediate reinjection protocol because of its time-saving and patient-convenient aspects. Besides, this approach provides at least similar information on myocardial perfusion and viability in patients with ischemic heart disease as the more established protocols [16,17]. Quantitative analysis of exercise and rest defect size by SPECT bulls-eye analysis enhances the confidence to distinguish patients with truly fixed defects from those with defect reversibility. Figure 1 shows the currently established protocols for ^{201}Tl myocardial perfusion imaging.

Myocardial imaging with ^{99m}Tc-sestamibi

One of the essential hallmarks of ^{99m}Tc-sestamibi is its lack of significant washout (or redistribution). Technetium-99m-sestamibi may be imaged well by planar scintigraphy, with or without electrocardiographic gating. However, the high photon flux it produces can be used with advantage with SPECT imaging. Myocardial images are usually of higher quality than those produced by ^{201}Tl scintigraphy. Because of the initially high liver uptake, which clears rapidly, the images are optimally acquired after 1 hour following ^{99m}Tc-sestamibi injection. Since ^{99m}Tc-sestamibi concentrates in the myocardium and does not undergo redistribution, two separate injections are required to distinguish stress-induced defects from resting defects.
The rest and stress images are ideally acquired on two different days to allow the decay of the initial activity to occur prior to the second injection [18]. This 2-day protocol allows injecting 20-30 mCi (750-1100 MBq) ^{99m}Tc-sestamibi during each of the 2 days. Alternatively, rest and exercise images may be acquired in the same day, using an initial dose of 10 mCi (370 MBq) followed by a second dose of 20 mCi (750 MBq). Taillefer et al.[19] have suggested that when two images acquired on the same day, the rest-stress protocol is somewhat superior to the stress-rest sequence, because some defects may appear to be reversible (ischemic) in the former protocol but fixed (scar) in the latter. However, when they compared the rest-stress with the stress-rest protocol, a concordance of 92% among normal, ischemic, or scarred segments was found; a discrepancy was observed in less than 8% of the myocardial segments analyzed. On the other hand, the advantage of performing the stress ^{99m}Tc-sestamibi images first is that is these stress images are normal, the rest images may not be necessarily, thus reducing in time for the study, the radiation dosimetry to the patient, and the cost of the study. The "ideal" protocol for ^{99m}Tc-sestamibi imaging will almost certainly need to be tailored to the individual institution's particular needs. For example, in an institution where patients with low likelihood of coronary artery disease are often imaged, a protocol beginning with the stress image first may be more cost- and time-effective,

since many of these patients will have a normal study, thus rendering the rest study redundant. If the stress studies are abnormal, a rest study ideally should be obtained on a separate day or several hours after the first injection.
The relative high dose of ^{99m}Tc can be used for assessment of global and regional left ventricular function. With a rapid bolus injection of ^{99m}Tc-sestamibi, first pass studies can be performed at rest and during exercise with specially designed high-count sensitive gamma cameras. The feasibility of using electrocardiographic gating for acquiring the myocardial images, with either planar or SPECT scintigraphy, improves the quality of the images by minimizing the motion of the heart [20]. Gated planar imaging is commonly performed by acquiring 16 frames per cardiac cycle. The images may subsequently be displayed in cine mode for wall motion and myocardial thickening assessment. Unfortunately, assessing wall motion and thickening may be difficult, especially in areas with decreased ^{99m}Tc-sestamibi uptake. A myocardial wall with diminished ^{99m}Tc-sestamibi uptake but with normal motion is probably viable. However, the concomitant occurrence of decreased wall motion and decreased uptake does not necessarily prove that the issue is nonviable, since both myocardial stunning and hibernating myocardium may be associated with hypoperfusion and hypokinesis. New computer techniques, albeit in the early stages of development, hold promise to quantitatively assess wall motion and thickening on sestamibi images.
Comparison of segmental perfusion by resting ^{99m}Tc-sestamibi images and wall motion by radionuclide angiography has been recently used to characterize myocardial viability [21]. In this study 77% of regions with normal or only mildly decreased perfusion (>50% of maximal uptake) were associated with either normal wall motion or mild hypokinesis by radionuclide angiography, indicating myocardial viability. Conversely, regions with severe hypoperfusion (<50% of maximal uptake) were usually associated with severe hypokinesis or akinesis, and hence were considered indicative of scarred myocardium. Furthermore, in this study 61% of segments with markedly reduced ^{99m}Tc-sestamibi uptake improved after coronary revascularization. Of the segments with mild to moderate hypoperfusion preoperatively (50% to 70% of maximal counts) 80% improved postoperatively, whereas only 39% of regions with ^{99m}Tc-sestamibi uptake less than 50% of maximal had significant improvement after revascularization.
In conclusion, best imaging results with ^{99m}Tc-sestamibi are obtained with the 2-day imaging protocol, because the count density of these images are usually excellent. From a more practical point of view a same-day protocol is preferred whereby stress imaging is performed first. The last option is more convenient for nuclear medicine laboratories, although one should be aware of relative low counts in the stress images. For simultaneous assessment of left ventricular perfusion and function ^{99m}Tc-sestamibi is the

imaging agent of choice. It can be anticipated that computer software will be developed that allows for quantitative assessment of myocardial perfusion, regional wall motion, and ejection fraction with one single image acquisition.

Dual-isotope imaging

In 1993, dual isotope imaging has been proposed as an alternative means for detecting CAD by Berman et al [22]. With this approach, ^{201}Tl is given at rest and ^{99m}Tc-sestamibi during stress. The protocol is a 1-day study whereby the patient is first injected at rest with 2.5-3.5 mCi (90-130 MBq) ^{201}Tl followed by imaging 15 minutes later. Immediately after completion of the rest imaging, stress imaging is performed with administration of 20-30 mCi ^{99m}Tc-sestamibi at peak exercise followed by imaging 30 minutes later. As this approach is significantly shorter than the same-day ^{99m}Tc-sestamibi protocols, this protocol was primarily designed to improve patient throughput. Although attractive from a practical point of view, disadvantages of the dual-isotope protocol are the use of ^{201}Tl at rest and the use of two tracers with different physical characteristics, affecting count density and imaging quality.

Myocardial imaging with ^{99m}Tc-teboroxime

The agent ^{99m}Tc-teboroxime is unique among myocardial perfusion agents because it has been shown a much better tracer of myocardial blood flow than ^{201}Tl or ^{99m}Tc-sestamibi [23]. However, the biokinetics of ^{99m}Tc-teboroxime are markedly different from those of ^{201}Tl and ^{99m}Tc-sestamibi in that is has a very rapid clearance from the myocardium. This characteristic of ^{99m}Tc-teboroxime precludes the acquisition of consistently good quality images, in particular when using SPECT imaging. Unless one employs specially designed fast-imaging protocols [24,25], clinical imaging with ^{99m}Tc-teboroxime is disappointing and the agent is therefore not widely used at the present time.

Myocardial imaging with ^{99m}Tc-tetrofosmin

Technetium-99m tetrofosmin is one of the most recently developed agents for myocardial perfusion imaging. Similar to ^{99m}Tc-sestamibi, ^{99m}Tc-tetrofosmin shows a very slow clearance from the myocardium allowing serial imaging during several hours. The ^{99m}Tc-tetrofosmin stress imaging protocol is based on the same-day ^{99m}Tc-sestamibi stress-rest protocol [26]. At peak stress 10 mCi (370 MBq) ^{99m}Tc-tetrofosmin is injected and imaging is started 15 minutes following termination of exercise. Three hours after the exercise injection, 20 mCi (750 MBq) is administered at rest followed by imaging 15 minutes later. The 15-minute period between injection and imaging is required because of liver activity and its subsequent clearance. A modification of this protocol, currently performed in the Netherlands, is a same-day rest-stress protocol. At rest 7 mCi (250 MBq) ^{99m}Tc-tetrofosmin is administered followed by imaging 30-45 minutes later. The stress dosage (20 mCi, 750 MBq) is given 120 minutes after the rest injection, and stress imaging is performed 30 minutes following injection of the radionuclide. In this way performed, the imaging procedure results in a total investigation time of around 3.5 hours. Similar to ^{99m}Tc-sestamibi, the use of ^{99m}Tc-tetrofosmin allows the acquisition of first pass and gated SPECT studies. At present there is only limited clinical experience with ^{99m}Tc-tetrofosmin, but initial results reported by Zaret et al. [3] are very promising.

Detection of coronary artery disease

A pooled analysis of the six largest studies evaluating ^{201}Tl exercise SPECT for the detection of CAD has recently been reported [28]. Coronary angiography was used as the reference standard for assessing the sensitivity of SPECT with a >50% stenosis considered significant. Specificity was based on whether patients had normal coronary arteriograms or a low predicted risk (<5%) for CAD. The overall sensitivity of SPECT for detecting CAD was 90% (range 81-98%) for the 1.042 patients analyzed - 99% in those patients with, and 85% in those without, prior infarction. Most patients with single vessel (83%) and virtually all patients with double (93%) and triple (95%) vessel disease were detected. Furthermore, two-thirds of patients with multivessel involvement were correctly identified as having multivessel disease. Of the 1.328 abnormal coronary arteries, 79% were detected, with sensitivity increasing to 88% for arteries with ≥70% stenosis.

The specificity of SPECT was 70% for the 239 patients with normal arteriograms, but increased to 89% for those with low predicted risk. The lower specificity in patients with normal arteriograms is related to post-test referral bias since, in general, more patients with abnormal images undergo coronary angiography. The high specificity (84%) of SPECT for detecting the 1.468 angiographically normal coronary arteries in this series, is consistent with the 89% specificity observed in patients with low predicted risk. When comparing the diagnostic power of ^{201}Tl to that of ^{99m}Tc-sestamibi, similar sensitivities and specificities have been found when planar imaging was used [29]. When SPECT imaging was used, similar sensitivities and only a trend to higher specificities with ^{99m}Tc-sestamibi were observed [30]. However, because of its superior imaging qualities compared to ^{201}Tl, one could make a strong case for using ^{99m}Tc-sestamibi SPECT in obese patients and in women with massive breast tissue. As with any technique, strict quality control is necessary to obtain good results. When performed properly, exercise SPECT is highly accurate for detecting the presence, extent and location of CAD in patients referred for evaluation of chest pain syndromes.

Role of pharmacologic stress

Despite the wide clinical utility of exercise perfusion scintigraphy, 25-30% of patients referred for imaging cannot perform adequate exercise which may significantly reduce sensitivity. This is particularly true in patients who terminate exercise early for noncardiac reasons, such as claudication from peripheral vascular disease or dyspnea form a primary pulmonary condition. Furthermore, even in patients who do develop transient perfusion abnormalities during submaximal exercise, the extent of the jeopardized myocardial risk zone may be significantly underestimated. In order to broaden the clinical availability of perfusion scintigraphy, the pharmacologic vasodilators, adenosine and dipyridamole, and more recently, dobutamine, have steadily gained acceptance as alternatives to exercise stress.
Dipyridamole is an indirect coronary vasodilator which inhibits the extracellular transport of the primary vasodilator, adenosine, into cells where the latter is rapidly deaminated and neutralized. Dipyridamole also inhibits the enzyme directly responsible for inactivation of adenosine (adenosine deaminase). Intravenously administered adenosine interacts with specific cell surface receptors to induce maximal hyperemia in most patients at doses of 140 mcg/kg/minute. Due to its exceedingly short half-life (<2 seconds), adenosine must be given as a constant intravenous infusion prior to radionuclide administration. Dobutamine is a beta-agonist which has both direct positive chronotropic and inotropic effects but indirectly induces arteriolar coronary vasodilation by markedly increasing myocardial oxygen demands.
Pharmacologic stressors induce perfusion defects primarily by altering regional coronary blood flow based on the intrinsic coronary flow reserve of a given vascular bed. During exercise, but particularly with pharmacologic stress, blood flow to the vascular bed of a normal coronary artery will increase by 3-4 fold, whereas flow through an epicardially stenosed artery may change minimally despite a maximal distal hyperemic response. Since the initial uptake of ^{201}Tl and ^{99m}Tc-based radiopharmaceuticals is flow-dependent within physiologic ranges, myocardial count activity will also be relatively greater in vascular beds with greater flow. If at least a two-fold difference in relative count activity occurs, a perfusion defect will result.

During exercise stress, heterogeneous coronary blood flow coupled with increasing myocardial oxygen demands will induce ischemia in most patients with CAD. Dobutamine will also elicit ischemia in most patients with severe coronary stenoses by markedly increasing myocardial contractility, heart rate and blood pressure. Dobutamine creates heterogeneous coronary flow but to a lesser extent than that observed with pharmacologic coronary vasodilators. Conversely, pharmacologic vasodilators infrequently elicit ischemia since they minimally increase the rate-pressure product. These differences in pharmacologic stressors are important to recognize when combining them with perfusion scintigraphy or echocardiography. Inducing heterogeneous blood flow is necessary for detecting CAD with perfusion scintigraphy but heterogeneity in flow sufficient to cause ischemia is required to detect regional wall motion abnormalities with echocardiography.

Pharmacologic stressors have been studied extensively for detecting CAD. The recommended protocol for intravenous dosing of dipyridamole is 0.56 mg/kg over a 4-minute period followed by radionuclide injection. This dose of dipyridamole induces maximal coronary hyperemia in some 80% of patients. The overall sensitivity reported with dipyridamole scintigraphy is approximately 89% with a specificity of 78% [31]. These values may even be improved by using dipyridamole in conjunction with low-level exercise, originally described by Laarman et al [32]. As with exercise scintigraphy, SPECT is notably better for detecting and localizing CAD than planar imaging.

Adenosine has been studied in well over 1.000 patients at doses of 140 mcg/kg/min. The reported sensitivity and specificity of adenosine SPECT are 90% and 89%. respectively, with excellent comparability to exercise [33]. Although the experience with dobutamine scintigraphy is limited, Hays et al. [34] reported a sensitivity and specificity of 86% and 90%, respectively, at a maximal dobutamine dose of 40 mcg/kg/min. Marwick et al. [35] compared dobutamine and adenosine echocardiography to sestamibi SPECT in 97 consecutive patients without prior infarction. Adenosine and dobutamine were infused up to peak doses of 180 and 40 mcg/kg/min, respectively. In this trial, adenosine and dobutamine SPECT had equivalent sensitivity (86% and 80%, respectively), and specificity (71% and 74%, respectively), whereas the sensitivity of adenosine echocardiography was inferior to SPECT with either stressor (58%, $P<0.001$). The sensitivity of dobutamine echocardiography, however, was comparably high at 85% with a specificity of 82%. Similar reports from other investigators indicate that dobutamine is a more rational choice with echocardiography than pharmacologic coronary vasodilators, whereas all three major pharmacologic stressor agents can be combined successfully with SPECT.

Assessment of risk

Myocardial perfusion imaging is invaluable for assessing risk in a wide spectrum of patients. A negative perfusion scan for ischemia has been consistently shown to predict a very low annual risk (<1%) for death or non-fatal infarction when combined with either exercise or pharmacologic stressors [36,37]. Conversely, patients with scintigraphically assessed ischemia are at considerably higher risk, which increases with the extent of hypoperfused myocardium. As shown in a recent study using quantitative exercise SPECT, patients with perfusion defects significantly increased risk for death or non-fatal infarction (25%) compared to those with smaller defects (5%, $p<0.001$) [38]. Furthermore, defect size contributed most to overall risk when compared to angiographic or treadmill data.

Perfusion scintigraphy is also commonly used to assess patient risk prior to noncardiac surgery [39]. Pooled data from over 2.000 patients studied with dipyridamole scintigraphy indicate that <2% of those with either a normal perfusion scintigram or only a fixed defect developed a postoperative event compared to 21% of patients who demonstrated scintigraphic ischemia. The positive predictive accuracy of scintigraphic ischemia increased with the extent of myocardial involvement.

The decision to perform scintigraphy preoperatively should be tailored to each individual patient. In patients without a prior cardiovascular history, clinical criteria can generally detect a low risk group where scintigraphy is not warranted. In patients with multiple cardiac risk factors, imaging may only be justified to better direct coronary revascularization procedures prior to surgery. However, in heterogenous populations where risk can vary considerably, perfusion scintigraphy is the most cost-effective approach for deciding who should have coronary angiography and possible revascularization prior to a major surgical procedure.

Exercise scintigraphy can accurately risk stratify patients after myocardial infarction and is of greater relative value than routine coronary angiography or submaximal exercise testing for discriminating low from high risk patients. This has also been shown using dipyridamole or adenosine stress. With adenosine SPECT a very low one year cardiac event rate in patients with small (<20%) nonischemic perfusion defects is observed. Conversely, risk progressively increases with larger perfusion defects and relatively greater ischemia. Thus, there is mounting evidence that defect size and the extent of ischemia accurately predict risk in a wide spectrum of patients with CAD. At the present time, precise risk analyses based on the extent of left ventricular involvement have only been reported using myocardial perfusion scintigraphy.

Evaluation of the effects of therapy

Thallium-201 scintigraphy can accurately assess temporal changes in myocardial ischemia after successful coronary angioplasty or bypass surgery. Scintigraphy is particularly advisable in patients who have a suboptimal dilation and should be performed two to four weeks post angioplasty when vascular reactivity has subsided. Patients with persistent ischemic defects after angioplasty are known to be at high risk for restenosis, whereas those without ischemia have a very low restenosis rate. The major advantage of perfusion imaging over the exercise electrocardiogram and other noninvasive techniques is its ability to localize ischemia to specific vascular beds. This is important since patients may have recurrent chest pain not only from coronary restenosis but also progression of CAD in arteries not previously dilated. In patients after bypass grafting, comparison of preoperative and postoperative studies is helpful for assessing the initial adequacy of revascularization and the postoperative study can also serve as a baseline agent which to compare subsequent studies if cardiac symptoms should recur.

Sequential myocardial perfusion scintigraphy has also been successfully used to assess the efficacy of anti-anginal medications both in patients with coronary artery spasm and, more recently, in those with fixed obstructive CAD. Agents that improve coronary blood flow will diminish exercise-induced ischemia, limit heterogeneity in myocardial perfusion and thereby reduce scintigraphic defects. It has been observed that transdermal nitroglycerin patches can significantly reduce exercise-induced scintigraphic ischemia compared to placebo. In fact, over one third of patients randomized to active therapy may show a $>10\%$ reduction in their absolute perfusion defect size over a one week treatment period. If the total extent of jeopardized myocardium defines risk, it is logical to assume that by reducing or eliminating perfusion defects prognosis should improve. Prospective randomized trials are still needed to prove this hypothesis.

Determining the functional significance of coronary artery lesions

The angiographic severity of a coronary artery stenosis does not necessarily predict an abnormality in myocardial blood flow at rest or during exercise [40]. Furthermore, although the vascular bed of the left anterior descending coronary artery is approximately twice that of the right or circumflex coronary arteries, the relative contribution of each coronary artery to global myocardial perfusion varies widely in any individual patient [41] Therefore, it is not surprising that a patient with triple vessel disease may do exceedingly well if there is no abnormality in myocardial perfusion during exercise or pharmacologic stress, whereas another patient with only single vessel disease but a large ischemic perfusion defect may be at high risk for death or nonfatal infarction. In this regard, perfusion scintigraphy can aid the clinician in interpreting the angiographic information and in formulating a therapeutic regimen.

Conclusions

Myocardial perfusion scintigraphy, by virtue of its extensive clinical validation and versatility, is presently the technique of choice for evaluating patients with known or suspected CAD. Precise quantification of perfusion defects with SPECT has further improved risk stratification and can provide an accurate serial assessment of patients following therapeutic interventions. The development of new perfusion tracers has considerably widened our scope in order to further explore the physiologic mechanisms of myocardial perfusion and viability. In conjunction with the application of vasodilatory substances, myocardial stress perfusion scintigraphy is now virtually accessible to all patients referred for cardiac evaluation. In this era of continuing cost containment, myocardial perfusion scintigraphy emerges as a highly cost effective noninvasive modality for guiding patient management.

References

1. Wackers FJ, Berman DS, Maddahi J, et al. Technetium-99m hexakis 2-methoxyisobutyl isonotrile: human biodistribution, dosimetry, safety, and preliminary comparison to thallium-201 for myocardial perfusion imaging. J Nucl Med 1989;30:301-11.
2. Zaret BL, Rigo P, Wackers FJT, et al. Myocardial perfusion imaging with ^{99m}Tc Tetrofosmin: comparison to ^{201}Tl imaging and coronary angiography in a phase III multicenter trial. Circulation 1995;91:313-9.
3. Verzijlbergen JF, Van Oudheusden D, Cramer MJ, et al. Quantitative analysis of planar technetium-99m sestamibi myocardial perfusion images. Clinical application of a modified method for the subtraction of tissue crosstalk. Eur Heart J 1994;15:1217-26.
4. Kiat H, Berman DS, Maddahi J. Comparison of planar and tomographic exercise thallium-201 imaging methods for the evaluation of coronary artery disease. J Am Coll Cardiol 1989;13:613-6.
5. Mahmarian JJ, Pratt CM, Borges-Neto S, et al. Quantification of infarct size by thallium-201 photon emission computed tomography during acute myocardial infarction. Circulation 1988;78:831-9.
6. Mahmarian JJ, Pratt CM, Nishimura S, et al. Quantitative adenosine Tl-201 single-photon emission computed tomography for the early assessment of patients surviving acute myocardial infarction. Circulation 1993;87:1197-210.
7. Kiat H, Berman DS, Maddahi J, et al. Late reversibility of tomographic myocardial thallium-201 defects: an accurate marker of myocardial viability. J Am Coll Cardiol 1988;12:1456-63.

8. Kayden DS, Sigal S, Soufer R, Mattera J, Zaret BL, Wackers FJ. Thallium-201 for assessment of myocardial viability: quantitative comparison of 24-hour redistribution imaging with imaging after reinjection at rest. J Am Coll Cardiol 1991;18:1480-86.
9. Dilzisian V, Rocco TP, Freeman NMT, Leon MB, Bonow RO. Enhanced detection of ischemic but viable myocardium by reinjection of thallium after stress redistribution imaging. N Engl J Med 1991;323:141-6.
10. Kuijper AFM, Vliegen HW, Van der Wall EE, et al. The clinical imact of thallium-201 reinjection scintigraphy for detection of myocardial viability. Eur J Nucl Med 1992;19;783-99.
11. Van Eck-Smit BLF, Van der Wall EE, Kuijper AFM, Zwinderman AH, Pauwels EKJ. Immediate thallium-201 reinjection following stress imaging: a time-saving approach for detection of myocardial viability. J Nucl Med 1993;34:737-43.
12. Wackers FJ, Pieri PL, McMahon M, et al. Quantitative reproducibility of repeated planar thallium stress imaging [abstract]. J Nucl Med 1993;34:44P.
13. He ZX, Darcourt J, Guignier A, et al. Nitrates improve detection of ischemic viable myocardium by thallium-201 reinjection SPECT. J Nucl Med 1993;34:1472-7.
14. Burns RJ, Galligan L, Wright L. Thallium infusion scintigraphy improves detection of viable myocardium [abstract]. Circulation 1990;82(suppl):III-554.
15. Ragosta M, Beller GA, Watson DD, et al. Quantitative planar rest-redistribution ^{201}Tl imaging in detection of myocardial viability and prediction of improvement in left ventricular function after coronary bypass surgery in patients with severely depressed left ventricular function. Circulation 1993;87:1630-41.
16. Van Eck-Smit BLF, Van der Wall EE, Zwinderman AH, Pauwels EKJ. Clinical value of immediate thallium-201 reinjection imaging for the detection of ischemic heart disease. Eur Heart J 1995;16:410-20.
17. Van Eck-Smit BLF, Van der Wall EE. Reinjection of thallium-201: why not immediate? Br Heart J. In Press.
18. Taillefer R, Laflamma L, Dupras G, Picard M, Phaneuf DC, Léveille J. Myocardial perfusion imaging with ^{99m}Tc-methoxy-isobutyl-isonitrile (MIBI): comparison of short and long time intervals between rest and stress injection. Eur J Nucl Med 1988;13:515-22.
19. Taillefer R. Technetium-99m sestamibi myocardial imaging: same-day stress-rest studies and dipyridamole Am J Cardiol 1990;80E-84E.
20. Verzijlbergen JF, Suttorp MJ, Ascoop CAPL, et al. Combined assessment of technetium-99m sestamibi planar myocardial perfusion images at rest and during exercise with rest-exercise left ventricular wall motion studies evaluated from gated myocardial perfusion studies. Am Heart J 1992;123:59-68.
21. Rocco TP, Dilsizian V, Strauss HW, Boucher CA. Technetium-99m isonitrile myocardial uptake at rest. II. Relation to clinical markers of potential viability. J Am Coll Cardiol 1989;14:1678-84.
22. Berman DS, Kiat H, Friedman JD, et al. Separate acquisition rest thallium-201/stress technetium-99m sestamibi dual isotope myocardial perfusion single photon emission computed tomography: a clinical validation study. J Am Coll Cardiol 1993;22:1455-64.
23. Seldin DW, Johnson LL, Blood DK, et al. Myocardial perfusion imaging with technetium SQ30217: comparison with thallium-201 and coronary anatomy. J Nucl Med 1989;30:312-319.
24. Hendel RC, McSherry B, Karimeddini M, Leppo JA. Diagnostic value of a new myocardial perfusion agent, teboroxime (SQ 30,217), utilizing a rapid planar imaging protocol: preliminary results. J Am Coll Cardiol 1990;16:855-861.
25. Chua T, Kiat H, Germano G, et al. Rapid back to back adenosine stress/rest technetium-99m teboroxime myocardial perfusion SPECT using a triple-detector camera. J Nucl Med 1993;34:1485-93.

26. Jain D, Wackers FJ, Mattera J, McMahon M, Sinusas AJ, Zaret BL. Biokinetics of ^{99m}Tc-tetrofosmin, a new myocardial perfusion imaging agent: implications for a one day imaging protocol. J Nucl Med 1993;34:1254-59.
27. Sridhara BS, Braat S, Rigo P, et al. Comparison of myocardial perfusion imaging with technetium-99m-tetrofosmin versus thallium-201 in coronary artery disease. Am J Cardiol 1993;72:1015-9.
28. Mahmarian JJ, Pratt CM, Boyce TM, Verani MS. The variable extent of jeopardized myocardium in patients with single vessel coronary artery disease: quantification by thallium-201 single photon emission computed tomography. J Am Coll Cardiol 1991;17:355-62.
29. Verzijlbergen JF, Cramer MJ, Niemeyer MG, et al. Tc99m-sestamibi for planar myocardial perfusion imaging;not as ideal as the physical properties. Nucl Med Commun 1991;12:381-91.
30. Cramer MJ, Verzijlbergen JF, Van der Wall EE, et al. Head-to-head comparison between technetium-99m sestamibi and thallium-201 tomographic imaging for the detection of coronary artery disease using combined dipyridamole exercise-stress. Coronary Artery Dis 1994;5:787-91.
31. Laarman GJ, Bruschke AVG, Verzijlbergen FJ, Bal ET, Van der Wall EE, Ascoop CAPL. Efficacy of intravenous dipyridamole with exercise in thallium-201 myocardial perfusion scintigraphy. Eur Heart J 1988;9:1206-14.
32. Laarman GJ, Niemeyer MG, Van der Wall EE, et al. Dipyridamole thallium testing: noncardiac side effects, cardiac effects, electrocardiographic changes and hemodynamic changes after dipyridamole infusion with and without exercise. Int J Cardiol 1988;20:231-8.
33. Nishimura S, Mahmarian JJ, Boyce TM, et al. Quantitative thallium-201 single-photon emissoin computed tomography during maximal pharmacologic coronary vasodilation with adenosine for assessing coronary artery disease. J Am Coll Cardiol 1991;18:736-45.
34. Hays JT, Mahmarian JJ, Cochran AJ, Verani MS. Dobutamine thallium-201 tomography for evaluating patients with suspected coronary artery disease unable to undergo exercise or vasodilator pharmacologic stress testing. J Am Coll Cardiol 1993;21:1583-90.
35. Marwick T, Willemart B, D'Hondt A, et al. Selection of the optimal nonexercise stress for the evaluation of ischemic regional myocardial dysfunction and malperfusion. Comparison of dobutamine and adenosine using echocardiography and ^{99m}Tc-MIBI single photon emission computed tomography. Circulation 1993;87:345-54.
36. Brown KA. Prognostic value of thallium-201 myocardial perfusion imaging. A diagnostic tool comes of age. Circulation 1991;83:363-81.
37. Oosterhuis WP, Breeman A, Niemeyer MG, et al. Patients with a normal exercise thallium-201 myocardial scintigram: always a good prognosis? Eur J Nucl Med 1993;20:151-8.
38. Iskandrian AS, Chae SC, Heo J, Stanberry CD, Wasserleben V, Cave V. Independent and incremental prognostic value of exercise single-photon emission computed tomographic (SPECT) thallium imaging in coronary artery disease. J Am Coll Cardiol 1993;22:665-70.
39. Eagle KA, Coley CM, Newell JB, et al. Combining clinical and thallium data optimizes preoperative assessment of cardiac risk before major vascular surgery. Ann Intern Med 1989;110:859-66.
40. White CW, Wright CB, Doty DB, et al. Does visual interpretation of the coronary arteriogram predict the physiologic importance of a coronary stenosis? N Engl J Med 1984;310:819-24.
41. Mahmarian JJ, Pratt CM, Boyce TM, Verani MS. The variable extent of jeopardized myocardium in patients with single vessel coronary artery disease: quantification by thallium-201 single photon emission computed tomography. J Am Coll Cardiol 1991;17:355-62.

Use of positron emission tomography for the diagnosis and evaluation of ischemic heart disease

Th.H. Marwick
Department of Cardiology, Cleveland Clinic International Center, U.S.A.

Summary

Positron emission tomography differs from conventional single photon techniques on the basis of basic physical principles, which translate into better image and contrast resolution, and avoidance of soft tissue attenuation. Consequently, PET is more accurate than SPECT. This is of value in myocardial perfusion imaging, particularly in obese patients, when questions are raised about physiological significance of mild coronary lesions, in complex patients, and in those with prior myocardial infarction. The accuracy of PET imaging for the diagnosis of coronary artery disease is about 90%. The physical principles of PET also favor a fully quantitative approach, which may be used to exactly measure myocardial blood flow. The other major indication of cardiac PET is the identification of viable myocardium, for which the most established technique is FDG imaging. This method is sensitive for the detection of viable myocardium but some variability in its specificity has been reported. New techniques which have been used to examine myocardial viability include evaluation of C-11 acetate clearance, quantitation of rubidium washout, and the perfusible tissue index. The examination of cardiac receptor status with PET may become clinically useful in the future.

Principles of positron emission tomography

Positron-emitting radionuclides are generally cyclotron-produced (though some may be derived from generators). These unstable compounds decay by release of a positron, or positively charged electron, which travels for a distance less than 1 cm before colliding with an electron. This collision causes the disintegration of both particles, with a

E. E. van der Wall et al. (eds.), Advances in Imaging Techniques in Ischemic Heart Disease 17–30.

resulting release of energy as two photons at 180^0 to each other [1]. Unlike the photons released by thallium (approximately 90 keV) or technetium (approximately 250 keV) these photons have an energy of 511 keV, and are less prone to be attenuated by overlying tissue structures than those arising from conventional radionuclides.

The positron scanner is comprised of several rims of detectors which surround the patient. Using an electronic coincidence detection mechanism, an "event" (positron release within the field of view of the scanner) may be defined by simultaneous activation of opposite detectors. This precludes the detection of photons which are scattered from other structures. As several rings of detectors surround the patient, a three-dimensional, transaxial image of the heart within the chest may be derived from these data [1]. Subsequently, the image is back-projected to obtain transverse, vertical and horizontal long axis views of the heart.

The benefits of positron emission tomography (PET) over conventional single photon (SPECT) techniques may be identified from the foregoing introduction. First, as PET tracers have a short half-life, their radiation dosimetry is more favorable than that of conventional isotopes, and more tracer can be administered. The use of short-acting tracers also permits the acquisition of true resting images of myocardial flow during myocardial perfusion imaging. The higher counts, together with the lower attenuation of high energy photons, means that many more counts are received by the detectors than during a conventional scintigraphic study. Not surprisingly, PET is about 10 times more sensitive than SPECT [2]. Better image quality and less partial volume effect are obtained with PET [2] as its spatial resolution is about 6-10 mm (compared with 10-15 mm for SPECT). The high counts obtained with PET permit the use of attenuation correction, and this methodology together with the use of high energy photons, avoids artifacts due to tissue attenuation. This in turn leads to more reliable imaging of the inferior wall, as well as the anterior wall in women [3].

Although PET has been used as a "noninvasive biochemical assay" to study many interesting processes in the heart (Table 1), it's current clinical application is limited to assessment of myocardial perfusion and myocardial viability.

Examination of myocardial perfusion using PET

The underlying principles of using PET for evaluation of myocardial perfusion are the same as with conventional techniques [4]. PET tracer is delivered to myocardium in proportion to regional perfusion; as blood flow increases during coronary hyperemia, the myocardial extraction of some tracers is reduced in a non-linear fashion and quantitative techniques for examining coronary flow or coronary flow reserve are

Table 1: Use of positron emission tomography to study cardiac blood flow and metabolic function.

Physiologic process	Tracer
Myocardial perfusion	Rb-82, N-13 ammonia, O-15 water, Cu-62 PTSM
Absolute myocardial blood flow	N-13 ammonia, O-15 water
Myocardial membrane function	Rb-82 washout
Fatty acid metabolism	C-11 palmitate
Exogenous glucose utilization	F-18 deoxyglucose
Oxidative phosphorylation	C-11 acetate
Myocardial hypoxia	F-18 misonidazole
Amino acid metabolism	Various N-13 or C-11 labelled amino acids
Receptor status	Various transmitters (mainly C-11 labelled)

dependent upon correction for this using a mathematical model. Four positron emitting tracers are used for myocardial perfusion studies: Rb-82, N-13 ammonia, O-15 water, and Cu-62 PTSM. Of these, the most convenient is Rb-82, as it permits the performance of PET using a generator rather than a cyclotron [5]. The half-life of Rb-82 is only 76 seconds, so that separate rest and stress images may be obtained independently in a short time-frame. The Rb-82 positron is of high energy and travels a long distance (about 1 cm) before undergoing an annihilation reaction: this gives a lower intrinsic resolution with Rb-82 than the other isotopes. N-13 ammonia is cyclotron-produced and has a half-life of 10 minutes; a period of 30-40 minutes is therefore required between the rest and stress injections. N-13 ammonia uptake is non-homogeneous in normal myocardium, with lower uptake in the lateral wall at rest and during stress [6]. While these physical aspects are less convenient than Rb-82, the myocardial uptake of N-13 ammonia is less effected by high flow rates and it is more attractive for quantitative purposes [7]. Cu-62 PTSM is also generator-produced, but the clinical experience with this compound is currently limited. O-15 water is ideal for quantitative flow measurement because it enjoys free diffusion across myocyte membranes and its retention is not influenced by ischemia. However, the performance of this approach for clinical purposes is unduly cumbersome, requiring substraction of cardiac blood pool tracer activity, and dynamic imaging [8].

While attenuation correction is an important strength of PET imaging, it does mandate the same positioning of the patient at rest and during stress. For this reason, PET perfusion imaging is generally performed with pharmacologic stress (dipyridamole or adenosine) in between the rest and stress images. The rubidium protocol entails an initial transmission scan of 10-15 minutes, a resting flow study over 5 minutes, pharmacologic stress (usually about 6 minutes), and a repeat perfusion study over 5 minutes [9]. Because of the longer half-life of N-13 ammonia, the total duration of studies with this compound is between 1-1/2 and 2 hours. However, the difficulties posed by exercise are a limitation of PET perfusion imaging, as in patients who are able to exercise, work capacity and ST segment response are well established as prognostically important parameters.

Table 2 summarizes the data on accuracy which has been obtained using PET for the detection of coronary artery disease. While the sensitivity and specificity have both been reported to be in the 90% range, these figures hide some important concerns. First, the total number of patients studied in all of these reports is less than 500, so that this experience is miniscule compared with the accuracy data available with SPECT or even stress echocardiography. Second, the critical question relating to the diagnostic use of PET is it's accuracy in patients without myocardial infarction, and all of the studies listed in Table 2 have included post-infarct patients, whose presence tends to augment the observed sensitivity of the study. Despite these reservations, PET has demonstrated a high sensitivity and specificity in localizing disease in the territory of the left anterior descending and right coronary arteries, being somewhat less effective in the circumflex territory, which probably reflects the heterogeneity of tissues supplied by the latter vessel [10].

Table 2: Sensitivity and specificity of positron emission tomography for the detection of significant (>50% stemosis) CAD (does not include studies related to other measures of stenosis severity).

Author	Tracer	n	MI (%of all)	Sensitivity	Specificity
Schelbert (Am J Cardiol 1982)	N-13	45	?	31/32 (97%)	13/13 (100%)*
Yonekura (Am Heart J 1987)	N-13	50	43%	37/38 (97%)	13/14 (93%)*
Tamaki (J Nucl Med 1988)	N-13	51	74%	47/48 (98%)	3/3 (100%)
Go (J Nucl Med 1990)	Rb-82	202	47%	142/152 (93%)	39/50 (78%)
Stewart (Am J Cardiol 1991)	Rb-82	81	42%	50/60 (84%)	19/21 (88%)
* Including normal volunteers					

Few data are available to guide the selection of PET in preference to SPECT. Of the three reported studies, the first, by Tamaki et al. reported similar sensitivities with both approaches, but involved a population with a high pre-test probability of disease [11].

The second involved a study of 202 patients at the Cleveland Clinic Foundation, which showed a significantly higher sensitivity of PET over SPECT with a comparable specificity. The reported specificity was lower than that obtained in other studies, which may in turn have reflected the inclusion of a broad spectrum of patients with cardiac pathology, including those with hypertrophy and valvular disease [9]. The third study of 81 patients found a higher specificity of PET in preference to SPECT with similar sensitivities but involved various stressors [12]. PET has proven more effective than SPECT in the detection of coronary disease after coronary bypass surgery [13]. Comparisons of diagnostic accuracy suggest that PET is somewhat more accurate than SPECT, although considering the cost of PET, the degree of benefit is not sufficient to recommend its routine use. Similarly, with respect to the accurate localization of coronary disease, PET has been found to be more accurate than SPECT. In a head-to-head comparison of PET and SPECT using the coronary angiogram as the arbitor of which test was correct, three important discrepancies emerged [14]. First, patients with moderate coronary stenoses, and those with coronary disease involving the posterior wall were more readily detected by PET than SPECT. Second, false positives due to soft tissue attenuation were less common with PET. Third, patients without a history of previous infarction were often found to have an apparent fixed perfusion defect by SPECT when PET demonstrated the presence of ischemia.

The causes of these discrepancies and the comparative data may be used to guide the selection of patients for PET rather than SPECT. First, because of the benefits of tissue attenuation, obese patients and females with large breasts are more readily studied with PET than SPECT. Second, because of the sensitivity for mild coronary disease and the superior localization of PET, studies being performed to identify a "culprit" coronary artery prior to coronary intervention may be better performed with PET than SPECT. Third, in patients with prior myocardial infarction, if for some reason reinjection thallium or delayed thallium imaging cannot be performed, perfusion defects may be more readily detected as reversible with PET than SPECT. Fourth, in patients with complicated coronary anatomy and prior myocardial infarctions, for example some patients being re-evaluated after coronary bypass surgery, the higher contrast and spatial resolution may produce more favorable results with PET than SPECT.

Quantification of myocardial blood flow

PET may be used to quantify myocardial blood flow, and blood flow measurements (in mls/minute/ 100 grams of myocardium) have been measured reproducibly with O-15 water [8,15,16] and N-13 ammonia [17-19]. However, this is technically more challenging than the use of PET for the diagnosis and localization of coronary disease, because dynamic acquisitions are required which are highly sensitive to patient motion. The uptake of tracer activity detected scintigraphically is entered into a sophisticated computer model of tracer biodistribution, usually derived from animal data, in order to obtain absolute blood flow.

Resting blood flow in normal healthy volunteers have been shown in studies using various radiotracers to range from 70-80 mls/minute/100 gram of tissue. Resting flow is influenced by the resting rate pressure product, and should probably be corrected for this [20]. In the presence of maximal coronary vasodilation, flow increases between 3 and 5 times, this variation reflecting differences in resting flow as well as driving pressure during maximal coronary hyperemia [21]. The clinical value of these quantitative blood flow measurements remains to be established; while severe coronary stenoses correlate closely with abnormal flow reserve, the correlation between coronary reserve and milder degrees of stenosis (50-70% diameter) is more variable. This may reflect the more "physiologic" data obtainable with PET, the results of which are influenced by collateral flow, for example. Whether subclassifying patients with more moderate stenoses based upon their flow reserve results permits the planning of more rational and effective treatment strategies remains to be defined. One interesting finding with this technology has been the detection of reduced flow reserve in apparently normal coronary vessels in patients with localized coronary stenosis in another territory [20]. The presence of this functionally abnormal vasculature may be indicative of early atherosclerotic changes in asymptomatic patients at risk of coronary disease, and quantitative PET may be useful for early detection of these patients and aggressive intervention with risk factor control [22].

Detection of viable myocardium using PET

It is now well recognized that following myocardial infarction, approximately 50% of dysfunctional segments are potentially recoverable [23]. Pathophysiologically, a number of explanations for this phenomenon are available. They include the presence of chronic ischemia, the presence of stunned myocardium, and that of hibernating myocardium. Stunned myocardium is characterized by post-ischemic dysfunction, which produces reduced contractility in the presence of normal resting flow [24]. Hibernating myocardium is classically defined as a state of down-regulation of the myocardium to produce less contractile function in the presence of reduced resting flow [25], although this tissue is not truly ischemic in the sense of showing normal metabolic hallmarks of ischemia, such as lactate production. In reality however, such segments are frequently comprised of various combinations of normal, ischemic, stunned, hibernating, and infarcted myocardium.

The conventional approaches for identifying the presence of infarcted myocardium include the presence of electrocardiographic Q waves, resting wall motion abnormalities, and persistent defects on standard 4 hour thallium redistribution images. Unfortunately however, none of these criteria reliably identify the presence of viable tissue [23]. The three current alternatives for this purpose are the use of dobutamine echocardiography (discussed in another chapter), other thallium protocols including reinjection and late redistribution (which identify viable tissue on the basis of an intact cell membrane which is able to concentrate thallium within the cell), and metabolic imaging using PET.

The most widely used PET technique for the detection of myocardial viability is one which examines the relative distribution of exogenous glucose utilization (with F-18 deoxyglucose, FDG) in relation to blood flow measured using the above tracers. FDG is closely analogous in structure to glucose, and crosses the capillary and myocyte membrane in a similar fashion. Following uptake into the cell, FDG is phosphorylated, but then becomes trapped in the cell as, unlike glucose, it is not a favorable substrate for glycolysis, glycogen synthesis, or the pentose phosphate shunt [26]. Thus, FDG uptake reflects the uptake of glucose into the cell rather than its subsequent metabolism. Cardiac myocytes normally utilize fatty acids for energy requirements, but glucose is normally utilized during ischemia or the post-prandial state [27]. Thus, the metabolic milieu of the cell has an important influence on FDG uptake, which may impact on the results of the test in diabetic patients as well as limiting the ability to standardize glucose uptake between individuals. In these situations, the use of insulin for diabetics with a high fasting blood sugar, or a euglycemic glucose-insulin clamp may be of value [28]. For clinical purposes, however, FDG imaging is usually performed after a glucose load, and imaging is delayed for 40 minutes after FDG injection to permit glucose to be concentrated within the cell and phosphorylated.

FDG images are processed in a similar way to perfusion images described above. They should be interpreted in conjunction with the perfusion images and three patterns may be observed. When regional myocardial perfusion and FDG are both absent or reduced to a similar degree, a "match pattern" is described. This has been subclassified into a transmural match, where the FDG and perfusion are absent or markedly reduced, or a non-transmural match, where the reduction is still commensurate but the degree of reduction is mild to moderate in severity. The latter pattern infers the presence of a mixture of viable and nonviable tissue. A "perfusion-metabolism mismatch" is characterized by a reduction in perfusion disproportionate to the level of FDG, which may be normal. This pattern of viable tissue in the context of reduced flow is consistent with the presence of hibernating myocardium. However, it should be remembered that the "match-mismatch" algorithm does not account for the presence of stunned myocardium, which will be characterized by normal flow and reduced function. Certainly, in the presence of collateral dependent myocardium, normal resting blood flow associated with a severely impaired flow reserve may produce resting dysfunction, presumably due to recurrent episodes of myocardial stunning [29]. The cells in these segments have been shown to be dedifferentiated, and may indicate the structural correlate of enhanced glucose utilization. Certainly they are characterized by loss of contractile machinery, numerous glycogen granules and small but ultrastructurally normal mitochondria [30].

The most appropriate "gold standard" for measuring the accuracy of the PET mismatch pattern for detection of viable myocardium is the comparison of regional function before and after revascularization (Table 3). These studies show that the predictive value of a negative test (ie. improvement of regional function after revascularization in the absence of FDG uptake) generally exceeds 80% and that of a positive test also exceeds 80%. However, this segmental analysis hides the fact that fewer than 150 patients have been followed up. Some of the heterogeneity in the reported studies pertains to the methodology of the test performance as well as its interpretation.

Table 3: Accuracy of FGD-PET imaging for identification of viable myocardium (segmental analysis).

Author	n (patients)	Segments	Viability (%)	Sensitivity	Specificity
Tillisch, N Engl J Med 1981	17	67	55%	35/37 (95%)	24/30 (80%)
Tamaki, J Nucl Med 1989	22	46	50%	18/23 (78%)	18/23 (78%)
Tamaki, Am J Card Imag 1991	11	56	71%	40/40 (100%)	6/16 (38%)
Marwick, Circulation 1992	16	85	41%	25/35 (71%)	38/50 (76%)
Lucignani, Eur J Nucl Med 1992	14	54	74%	37/40 (93%)	12/14 (86%)
Carrel, Eur J Cardioth Surg 1992	21	23	74%	16/17 (94%)	3/6 (50%)
Gropler, J Am Coll Cardiol 1992	16	53	45%	19/24 (79%)	24/29 (83%)

Studies which have involved fasting or post-exercise FDG imaging may be used to detect ischemia as well as hibernating myocardium, and consequently may have a lower positive predictive accuracy for recovery of left ventricular dysfunction [31]. In respect of interpretation, the original approach normalized the FDG uptake to the myocardial segments which demonstrated > 90% of peak tracer concentration and defined "match" and "mismatch" by differences between FDG and perfusion. An alternate approach has been to normalize both perfusion and FDG to their respective highest concentrations and then evaluate the segmental ratios of FDG to perfusion [32]. This latter approach has been reported to have a low positive predictive value, although this may also pertain to the inclusion of segments with milder degrees of regional contractile dysfunction, in which circumstance the mismatch pattern may reflect the presence of non transmural infarction. Finally, quantitative analysis of glucose uptake without comparison to perfusion has shown a positive predictive accuracy of 70% and a negative predictive accuracy of 93% for prediction of subsequent functional recovery after revascularization [33]. As FDG has a much longer half-life than the PET perfusion tracers, it may be obtained in institutions without a cyclotron from a separate radiopharmacy, and comparitive perfusion scans may be obtained using SPECT isotopes (technetium MIBI or thallium). These hybrid imaging strategies are feasible and offer favorable findings. Finally, preliminary results obtained using FDG with SPECT imaging (using heavy collimators) has shown that this "poor man's metabolic study" may be able to provide similar levels of accuracy when PET is not available.

The detection of viable myocardium is clinically important on two grounds. First, if sufficient viable myocardium is present, left ventricular function may benefit from revascularization (Table 4).

Table 4: Response of ejection fraction (EF) to revascularization of viable myocardium.

Author	n (patients)	EF (pre)	EF (post)
Tillisch, N Engl J Med 1981	17	30±11	45±15
Marwick, Am J Cardiol 1992	16	37±11	40±19
Lucignani, Eur J Nucl Med 1992	14	38±5	48±4
Carrel, Eur J Cardioth Surg 1992	21	34±14	52±11
Vanoverschelde, Circulation 1993	11	55±7	65±8
Besozzi, J Nucl Med 1992	49	29±12	41±11

Indeed, using the post-exercise technique, which identifies both ischemic and viable tissue, increased FDG uptake in >20% of the left ventricle was associated with significant improvement of functional capacity of the patient [7]. Second, it has become apparent that the presence of non-revascularized viable tissue is associated with a disproportionate incidence of major subsequent cardiac events, while its revascularization is associated with a substantially lower event rate (Table 5). This observation may reflect two phenomena. First, "viable tissue" may represent incomplete infarction, with residual jeopardized tissue which is prone to reinfarction. Second, as the annual mortality of post-infarct patients has been shown to correlate with the severity of the left ventricular dysfunction [34], measures which improve left ventricular dysfunction could be expected to reduce mortality. In the current environment of limited numbers of donor hearts, cardiac transplantation may improve the survival in only a relatively small group of heart failure patients. On the other hand, PET may identify patients with ischemia and viability whose functional capacity and prognosis may be improved by simple revascularization rather than transplantation [35, 36]. In spite of the costs of PET, its accuracy in prediction of viable myocardium may make it cost effective for decision making regarding surgical therapy. Obviously, assessment of the extent of viable tissue, and therefore the likely degree of benefit are of vital importance in the situation where myocardial revascularization may be attended by a substantial mortality [36].

Table 5: Relationship between event-rate, revascularization decision (RVS) and viability by PET.

Author	Total (pts)	RVS decision incompatible with PET		RVS decision compatible with PET		Events
		Pts	Event-rate	Pts	Event-rate	
Di Carli, Am J Cardiol 1993	93	34 (37%)	8/34 (24%)	59 (63%)	6/59 (10%)	Death
Eitzman, J Am Coll Cardiol 1992	82	32 (39%)	10/32 (31%)	50 (61%)	6/50 (12%)	Ischemia, infarction, death
Yoshida, J Am Coll Cardiol 1993	35	9 (26%)	2/9 (22%)	26 (74%)	5/26 (19%)	Death
Lee, Circulation 1994	129	40 (31%)	14/40 (35%)	89 (69%)	15/89 (17%)	Ischemia, infarction, death

New techniques for the assessment of myocardial viability

While the FDG metabolism perfusion mismatch has been by far the most frequently used PET technique for identification of viable myocardium, in current clinical use, it is semi-quantitative, and attempts to quantitate it more accurately have been limited by the need to standardize the metabolic status of patients. Several alternative approaches may offer a more quantitative approach in this area. Probably the best investigated is the use of C-11 acetate to investigate the status of oxidative metabolism within the cell. C-11 acetate clearance has been shown to be significantly reduced in irreversibly dysfunctional segments, but is preserved in segments with reversible dysfunction [37]. Indeed, comparisons between C-11 acetate clearance and FDG metabolism-perfusion mismatch have suggested acetate to be a more accurate predictor of regional functional recovery [37]. However, other centers have documented a close correlation between C-11 acetate clearance (and hence oxidative metabolism) and absolute myocardial blood flow. On these grounds, it may be expected that acetate criteria would not be able to discern hibernating tissue. For similar reasons, while threshold levels of myocardial perfusion have been roughly predictive of viability, the interpretation of patients with intermediate levels of perfusion impairment can only be made with the addition of a metabolic tracer.

Two other approaches have focused on data supplementary to that gathered during perfusion imaging. As cation retention within the cell is an active process which requires an intact sodium potassium pump in the cell membrane, the ability of cells to retain tracer may be used as an indicator of myocardial viability. This is analogous to the mechanism through which thallium may be used for viability assessment, and some experience for this purpose has been gathered by examining rubidium washout, using dynamic imaging with a camera which is able to deal with high rubidium count rates. Preliminary data have shown favorable comparisons with the FDG approach [38]. A second perfusion-related approach to the determination of myocardial viability has been the use of the perfusible tissue index [39]. This analysis incorporates the tissue density obtained during routine transmission images. After correcting for blood volume in the myocardium by subtraction of images obtained using O-15 carbon monoxide within red cells, the resultant image portrays the extravascular tissue density. The fraction of this tissue which is able to exchange O-15 labelled water is the perfusible tissue index, which by definition involves only viable myocytes rather than scar tissue or necrotic cells. Preliminary results suggest that a perfusion tissue index of >0.7 is predictive of post revascularization improvement of contractile function, while an index of < 0.7 is associated with no improvement following revascularization.

Conclusion

Despite the expense of PET, this technique has important clinical potential in several areas. As the cost of revascularization procedures is about ten times that of PET imaging, the use of this test is cost efficient if revascularization decisions may be altered by the presence or absence of myocardial viability in patients with left ventricular dysfunction. Certainly, if cardiac transplantation is being considered, the cost of PET is small in comparison to the savings engendered by revascularization of patients with jeopardized myocardium. With respect to myocardial perfusion imaging, PET may be cost efficient if limited to subgroups of patients who are difficult to image by other means. Generally, this constitutes a small proportion of patients overall, and

PET facilities can be justified in large cardiology centers on these grounds. Finally, the role of PET as a "noninvasive biochemical assay" ensures its continued research use in studies of cardiac perfusion, metabolism and neurochemistry.

References

1. Bacharach SL. The physics of positron emission tomography. In: Bergmann SR, Sobel BE, editor. Positron emission tomography of the heart. Mount Kisco: Futura Publishing Company, 1992:13-44.
2. Koeppe RA, Hutchins GD. Instrumentation for positron emission tomography: tomographs and data processing and display systems. Sem Nucl Med 1992;22:162-81.
3. Eisner RI, Tamas MJ, Cloninger K, et al. Normal SPECT thallium-201 bulls-eye display: Gender differences. J Nucl Med 1988;29:1901-9.
4. Gould KL. Noninvasive assessment of coronary stenoses by myocardial perfusion imaging during pharmacologic coronary vasodilation. 1. Physiologic basis and experimental validation. Am Cardiol 1978;41:267-78.
5. Gould KL, Goldstein RA, Mullani NA, et al. Noninvasive assessment of coronary stenoses by myocardial perfusion imaging during pharmacologic coronary vasodilation. VIII. Clinical feasibility of positron cardiac imaging without a cyclotron using generator-produced rubidium-82. Am Coll Cardiol 1986;7:775-89.
6. Hutchins GD, Beanlands RS, Muzik O, Schwaiger M. Quantitative vs semi-quantitative PET myocardial blood flow: influence of regional ammonia kinetics [abstract]. Circulation 1992;86(4 suppl):I710.
7. Laubenbacher C, Rothley J, Sitomer J, et al. An automated analysis program for the evaluation of cardiac PET studies: initial results in the detection and localization of coronary artery disease using nitrogen-13-ammonia. J Nucl Med 1993;34:968-78.
8. Bergmann SR, Herrero P, Markham J, et al. Noninvasive quantitation of myocardial blood flow in human subjects with oxygen-15-labelled water and positron emission tomography. J Am Coll of Cardiol 1989;14:639-52.
9. Go RT, Marwick TH, MacIntyre WJ, et al. A prospective comparison of rubidium-82 PET and thallium-201 SPECT myocardial perfusion imaging utilizing a single dipyridamole stress in the diagnosis of coronary artery disease. J Nucl Med 1990;31:1899-905.
10. Schwaiger M. Myocardial perfusion imaging with PET. Journal of Nuclear Medicine. 1994;35:693-8.
11. Tamaki N, Yonekura Y, Senda M, et al. Value and limitation of stress thallium-201 single photon emission computed tomography: comparison with nitrogen-13 ammonia positron tomography. J Nucl Med 1988;29:1181-9.
12. Stewart RE, Schwaiger M, Molina E, et al. Comparison of rubidium-82 positron emission tomography and thallium-201 SPECT imaging for detection of coronary artery disease. Am J Cardiol 1991;67:130-3-10.
13. Marwick TH, Lafont A, Go RT, Underwood DA, Saha GB, MacIntyre WJ. Identification of recurrent ischemia after coronary artery bypass surgery: a comparison of positron emission tomography and single photon emission computed tomography. Int J Cardiol 1992;35:33-41.
14. Marwick TH, Go RT, MacIntyre WJ, Saha GB, Underwood DA. Myocardial perfusion imaging with positron emission tomography and single photon emission computed tomography: frequency and causes of disparate results. Eur Heart J 1991;12:1064-9.

15. Araujo LI, Lammertsma AA, Rhodes CG, et al. Noninvasive quantification of regional myocardial blood flow in coronary artery disease with oxygen-15-labeled carbon dioxide inhalation and positron emission tomography. Circulation 1991;83:875-85.
16. Uren NG, Melin JA, De Bruyne B, Wijns W, Baudhuin T, Camici P. Relation between myocardial blood flow and the severity of coronary artery stenosis. N Engl J Med 1991;330:1782-8.
17. Hutchins GD, Schwaiger M, Rosenspire KC, Krivokapich J, Schelbert HR, Kuhl DE. Noninvasive quantification of regional blood flow in the human heart using N-13 ammonia and dynamic positron emission tomographic imaging. J Am Coll Cardiol 1990;15:1032-42.
18. Czernin J, Muller P, Chan S, et al. Influence of age and hemodynamics on myocardial blood flow and flow reserve. Circulation 1993;88:62-9.
19. Muzik O, Beanlands RS, Hutchins GD, Mangner TJ, Nguyen N, Schwaiger M. Validation of nitrogen-13-ammonia tracer kinetic model for quantification of myocardial blood flow using PET. J Nucl Med 1993;34:83-91.
20. Uren NG, Marraccini P, Gistri R, De Silva R, Camici PG. Altered coronary vasodilator reserve and metabolism in myocardium subtended by normal arteries in patients with coronary artery disease. J Am Coll Cardiol 1993;22:650-8.
21. Gould KL, Kirkeeide RL, Buchi M. Coronary flow reserve as a physiologic measure of stenosis severity. J Am Coll Cardiol 1990;15:459-74.
22. Dayanikli F, Grambow D, Muzik O, Mosca L, Rubenfire M, Schwaiger M. Early detection of abnormal coronary flow reserve in asymptomatic men at high risk for coronary artery disease using positron emission tomography. Circulation 1994;90:808-17.
23. Brunken R, Tillisch J, Schwaiger M, et al. Regional perfusion, glucose metabolism, and wall motion in patients with chronic electrocardiographic Q wave infarctions: evidence for persistence of viable tissue in some infarct regions by positron emission tomography. Circulation 1986;73:951-63.
24. Kloner RA, Przyklenk K, Patel B. Altered myocardial states: The stunned and hibernating myocardium. Am J Med 1986;86:14-22.
25. Rahimtoola SH. The hibernating myocardium. Am Heart J 1989;117:211-21.
26. Phelps ME, Hoffman EJ, Selin C, et al. Investigation of [F-18] 2-fluoro-2-deoxyglucose for the measure of myocardial glucose metabolism. J Nucl Med 1978;19:1311-9.
27. Camici P, Ferrannini E, Opie LH. Myocardial metabolism in ischemic heart disease: Basic principles and application to imaging by positron emission tomography. Prog Cardiovasc Dis 1989;32:217-38.
28. Knuuti MJ, Nuutila P, Ruotsalainen U, et al. Euglycemic hyperinsulinemic clamp and oral glucose load in stimulating myocardial glucose utilization during positron emission tomography. J Nucl Med 1992;33:1255-62.
29. Vanoverschelde JL, Wijns W, Depre C, et al. Mechanisms of chronic regional postischemic dysfunction in humans. New insights from the study of noninfarcted collateral-dependent myocardium. Circulation 1993;87:1513-23.
30. Maes A, Flameng W, Nuyts J, et al. Histological alterations in chronically hypoperfused myocardium. Correlation with PET findings. Circulation 1994;90:735-45.
31. Marwick TH, MacIntyre WJ, Lafont A, Nemec JJ, Salcedo EE. Metabolic responses of hibernating and infarcted myocardium to revascularization. A follow-up study of regional perfusion, function, and metabolism. Circulation 1992;85:1347-53.
32. Gropler RJ, Geltman EM, Sampathkumaran K, et al. Functional recovery after coronary revascularization for chronic coronary artery disease is dependent on maintenance of oxidative metabolism. J Am Coll Cardiol 1992;20:569-77.

33. Knuuti MJ, Nuutila P, Ruotsalainen U, et al. The value of quantitative analysis of glucose utilization in detection of myocardial viability by PET. J Nucl Med 1993;34:2068-75.
34. Alderman EL, Fisher LD, Litwin P, et al. Results of coronary artery surgery in patients with poor left ventricular function (CASS). Circulation 1983;68:785-95.
35. Dreyfus G, Duboc D, Blasco A, et al. Coronary surgery can be an alternative to heart transplantation in selected patients with end-stage ischemic heart disease. Eur Cardiothorac Surg 1993;7:482-7, discussion 488.
36. Louie HW, Laks H, Milgalter E, et al. Ischemic cardiomyopathy. Criteria for coronary revascularization and cardiac transplantation. Circulation 1991;84(5 suppl):290-5.
37. Gropler RJ, Geltman EM, Sampathkumaran K, et al. Comparison of carbon-11-acetate with fluorine-18-fluorodeoxyglucose for delineating viable myocardium by positron emission tomography. J Am Coll Cardiol 1993;22:1587-97.
38. Gould L, Yoshida K, Hess M, et al. Myocardial metabolism of fluorodeoxyglucose compared to cell membrane integrity for the potassium analog rubidium-82 for assessing infarct size in man by PET. J Nucl Med 1991;32:1-9.
39. De Silva R, Yamamoto Y, Rhodes CG, et al. Preoperative prediction of the outcome of coronary revascularization using positron emission tomography. Circulation 1992;86:1738-42.

Magnetic resonance coronary angiography

P.M.T. Pattynama and A. de Roos
Department of Diagnostic Radiology and Nuclear Medicine, University Hospital Leiden, the Netherlands

Summary

Over the past few years, magnetic resonance (MR) angiography has rapidly evolved up to the point that it now becomes feasible to image the coronary arteries. A noninvasive method to assess the coronary arteries would be a clinically valuable asset. The technical demands for imaging the coronary arteries, however, are huge, considering the cardiac and respiratory motions and the small size of the vessels. To date, MR angiography can only visualize the proximal portions of the coronary tree and the larger sized venous aortocoronary bypasses. The accuracy to detect significant stenoses is as yet insufficient. This may change, however, in the near future with implementation of echoplanar imaging, dedicated phased array surface coils and intravenously administered MR blood pool markers. It is hoped that MR coronary angiography, now an experimental method, will further mature into a method for reliable noninvasive imaging of coronary artery morphology and function.

Introduction

At several stages of ischemic heart disease it is important to evaluate the coronary arteries. In chronic angina, the site and severity of coronary stenoses are important risk factors of developing infarction. After myocardial infarction, the patency of the infarct-related artery is a major prognostic factor [1], and after coronary surgery, follow-up studies are indicated to assess the status of the coronary bypasses. Conventional X-ray angiography is the time-honored method to depict the coronary vessels. Over the past few years, other modalities have emerged which potentially are capable of doing the same. A particularly attractive technique is magnetic resonance (MR) angiography, which is noninvasive and requires no ionizing radiation or iodinated contrast media.

E. E. van der Wall et al. (eds.), Advances in Imaging Techniques in Ischemic Heart Disease 31–45.

This article reviews the principles of MR angiography and its current status for imaging the coronary arteries.

Ever since the early days of clinical MR imaging it has been known that protons (spins) in flowing blood differ from those in static tissue. Flowing blood often causes disturbing artifacts in the MR images. Large research efforts have been made not just to mitigate these unwanted flow artifacts, but even to use these artifacts to better advantage. Imaging pulse sequences were designed that on the one hand enhanced the flow effects while on the other hand suppressed signal from the nonmoving, stationary tissues. In the resulting MR images the flowing blood stands out from its surroundings: MR angiography. The MR data can be displayed as images that somewhat resemble conventional X-ray angiograms. The two methods, however, assess two fundamentally different features of flowing blood. The MR angiogram images blood flow, whereas conventional coronary angiography visualizes the vessel lumen. A severe reduction in the vessel diameter may be seen in MR angiography as a long complete "occlusion", because of signal loss in the region with poststenotic turbulent flow. MR angiography has the potential, aside from providing images of the blood vessels, to also measure the volume flow through the vessel. The sub-modality of MR angiography which addresses functional flow measurements is called flow mapping. For an understanding of the potential of MR angiography and also of its limitations and potential pitfalls, we will first discuss the flow effects that underly the image contrast in MR angiography.

Flow effects in MR angiography

There are two different flow effects that may be used to distinguish between flowing blood and stationary tissue. These phenomena are 1. Time-of-Flight (TOF) effects and 2. velocity-related phase changes (phase contrast, PC), and they provide the image contrasts that are used in TOF MR angiography and PC MR angiography, respectively.

Time-of-flight effects

For MR image formation, a given imaging slice is excited repeatedly with repetitive slice-selective radiofrequency pulses. In MR angiography, the period in between the pulses, the repetition time, is made very short, less than 30 msec. Stationary spins will experience all the repetitive pulses and do not have the time to recover during the short interval between two subsequent pulses. As a result, they remain strongly saturated with recovery of little available signal for imaging. The short repetition time thus results in stationary tissues with low signal intensity in the final MR image. By contrast, flowing spins that enter the imaging slice during image acquisition have not undergone previous excitation pulses. The magnetization of these "fresh" unsaturated spins is maximal which leads to high signal intensity. This is called the inflow refreshment, or Time-of-Flight phenomenon. When the flowing spins leave the imaging slice they will still contribute to the high intravascular signal. The imaging signal is acquired by a process called refocussing and this procedure is not slice-selective but is applied to the entire volume of examination. In the resulting MR image then, flowing blood will appear bright relative to a low signal intensity background. There exists a relationship between blood flow velocity and signal intensity. At low flow velocities, only few fresh spins enter the imaging plane and signal intensity will be low. With increasing velocities, more and more fresh spins enter the imaging slice with higher resultant signal intensity. The signal intensity within the vessel is maximal when all spins in the slice are completely replaced during the interval between two pulses, i.e., at a certain value of the flow velocity.

Phase contrast effects

Whereas TOF effects deal with the magnitude of the imaging signal, the phase contrast effects considers the phase of the signal. Whenever an excitation pulse is applied, the spins are forced to have the same phase and start to precess (rotate like a top) with a frequency that is proportional to the strength of the local magnetic field; they will precess faster in stronger than in weaker parts of the magnetic field. Phase differences (i.e., phase contrasts) between stationary and flowing spins can be evoked by briefly applying a bipolar gradient, a small magnetic field gradient along the expected direction of flow followed by an equal but opposite gradient. Dictated by the bipolar gradient, the spins will precess with different frequencies at different points in time and in space. Spins in stationary tissue experience an initial increase in precessing frequency. This effect is nullified by the second inverted gradient which temporarily slows down the spins. Flowing spins, however, because of their movement along the gradient through different field strengths, have precessed faster or slower than spins in stationary tissue, and their phase offset will not be nullified by the inverted gradient. They will thus obtain a net phase shift relative to stationary spins. The presence of a phase shift then distinguishes flowing blood from stationary tissue and this provides the contrast between blood vessels and stationary tissue in PC MR angiography.

The PC flow effect also forms the basis for the flow velocity measurements of MR flow mapping. The magnitude of the phase shifts is directly proportional to the spin velocity and can be measured accurately. The PC data can be used to create a phase map which can be translated into a velocity map, which is a spatial representation of the velocities within the imaging plane at the time of data acquisition. Because the blood flow is pulsatile, the velocity map changes over the course of the cardiac cycle. The MR data sampling is therefore triggered to the R-wave of the electrocardiogram. Velocity maps are obtained at 16 or more consecutive time points which together span the entire cardiac cycle. The functional flow data can be represented in many different ways, e. g. as a velocity map showing the spatial flow profile or as a time-flow diagram. The volume blood flow through the vessel per cardiac cycle is given by the area under the time-volume curve.

One of the advantages of MR flow mapping is that it can cover a wide range of flow velocities, from 1 cm/sec to several hundreds of cm/sec. For optimal results, it is necessary to adjust the system for the velocity range one wishes to consider. This is done by adjusting the magnitude of the bipolar gradient that brings about the PC effects. Application of the bipolar gradient (velocity encoding) can be done in any direction, but is often performed in only one direction, e.g. perpendicular to the imaging plane. The method can be extended by applying velocity encoding in three orthogonal planes. This allows the three-dimensional (3D) evaluation of the magnitude and direction of the spin velocities, but only at the expense of doubling the acquisition time.

Comparison of TOF and PC MR angiography

A discussion of the relative advantages of TOF versus PC MR angiography is outside the scope of this chapter and can be found in review articles [2,3]. Some characteristics of the two methods, though, deserve mentioning. Common to both techniques is the need for short repetition times and short echo times. Short repetition times, as was already mentioned, reduce the signal from stationary tissue. Short echo times are required to maintain a high vascular signal. A significant reduction of MR signal is caused by loss of phase coherence inside each voxel, an effect that occurs especially when the voxel contains spins with many different velocities. If there is loss of phase coherence, the net magnetization is zero and signal is lost. This effect tends to exaggerate the severity of the stenosis, e.g. by causing signal loss in regions of poststenotic turbulence. This artifact is counteracted by reducing the echo time between excitation and signal read-out which will leave the spins with less time to dephase. Phase dispersion is further decreased by minimizing the voxel size (e.g. by using thin slices). This has the effect of increasing the number of voxels that each have more homogeneous velocity distributions.

In TOF MR angiography, all vessels entering the imaging slice will appear bright, irrespective of the flow direction. It may at times thus be difficult to distinguish between arteries and veins. Signal from either of the two can be suppressed with a presaturation slab that is applied on one side of the imaging plane. Spins flowing from the presaturation slab into the imaging slice will be presaturated and will not contribute signal. In the resulting MR angiogram, that particular vessel will not be seen. From the description of the inflow phenomenon it follows that vessel segments coursing within the imaging plane for some distance will not be imaged well: the spins will become saturated by the repetitive excitation pulses. Spin saturation with loss of imaging signal will also present a problem when the imaging section (or volume) is made too thick. Another drawback of the TOF method is that low flow is not imaged very well.

PC MR angiography has several advantages over the TOF technique. The background suppression is usually very good. Imaging of thick (several cm) slices will not cause signal loss and may in fact be used for clinically useful projection images (see below). Also, imaging of slow flow can be accomplished by selecting the appropriate velocity range. Disadvantages of the PC method include longer acquisition times. At present, TOF MR angiography is the more widely used technique. It may well be that this will change with technical improvements, considering the advantage of the PC method of providing measurements of volume flow.

Imaging modes and image display

To obtain useful MR angiograms, multiple contiguous imaging slices are required that cover the vessel segment under consideration. Both TOF and PC MR angiography can be applied in two-dimensional (2D) or 3D imaging modes. In the 2D mode, multiple single thin slices are imaged one after the other, whereas in the 3D mode, an entire volume is imaged as a whole and later divided into thin sections. Both the 2D techniques [4] and 3D techniques [5] have been used for MR coronary angiography. Although still preliminary, new projectional techniques appear to be promising for use with MR coronary angiography. A single projection of flow in the coronary arteries is obtained by imaging a volume of interest which contains the vessel of interest [6,7].

Adequate presentation of the large amount of imaging data is essential for proper interpretation of the MR examinations. The first reprojection technique that has been developed, and also the most widely used in MR angiography, is the maximum-intensity-projection method [8]. With this algorithm, the brightest pixels along a user-defined direction are extracted to create a projection image. An unlimited number of projections can be acquired from any desired direction from a single data set, including projection normally not feasible with conventional angiography. Projection images obtained at small (3-5 degrees) intervals can be rapidly displayed sequentially in a cine-loop mode, and this allows a better appreciation of the 3D relationship between the vessels. The maximum-intensity-projection display, though, has several recognized deficiencies [9], e.g., overlapping vessels will be displayed as if they were branching vessels. Several research groups are experimenting with improvements on the maximum-intensity-projection display, e.g. by using 3D shaded surface rendering to add a sense of depth (Figure 1) or by making the projected vessels have more of the familiar characteristics of conventional angiograms, by increasing the intensity when the vessels overlap. It may well be that as full 3D display consoles become available the preferred method may be to rapidly scan through the images following the vessel's cross section.

Imaging the coronary arteries: a particular challenge

MR angiography of the coronary arteries is one of the most challenging areas in MR imaging. Substantial technical obstacles must be overcome. There are the respiratory and cardiac motions that tend to blur the images. Furthermore, the coronary arteries are small (3-5 mm in the proximal segments) and tortuous, which pose problems with regard to spatial resolution and signal-to-noise ratio (SNR). Overcoming all of these problems is currently beyond the technical limits even of the most dedicated cardiac MR systems. MR coronary angiography requires dedicated MR hardware and software and postprocessing, to date not available on commercial MR systems. MR coronary angiography is therefore performed in a limited number of MR research centers worldwide. The standard MR images only occasionally show portions of the coronary arteries, and MR angiography of the coronary arteries has only recently become feasible with the development of a new group of ultrafast imaging sequences. These newer sequences, it should be added, can be applied not only to MR angiography but also to MR flow mapping [10].

To overcome cardiac motion, the MR data acquisition is triggered to the electrocardiogram, at the expense of a prolonged imaging time. To cope also with respiratory motion, one might apply additional respiratory gating, but this would result in unacceptably long imaging times. Current efforts therefore focus on the use of the ECG-gated ultrafast MR sequences with complete data acquisition of the entire volume of interest within approximately 16 heartbeats. This allows, in a cooperative subject, completion of data acquisition within a single breath-hold. Suitable ultrafast MR imaging sequences now include speeded-up versions of the gradient-echo technique, and modifications of echo-planar imaging (EPI) [reviewed in: 11,12].

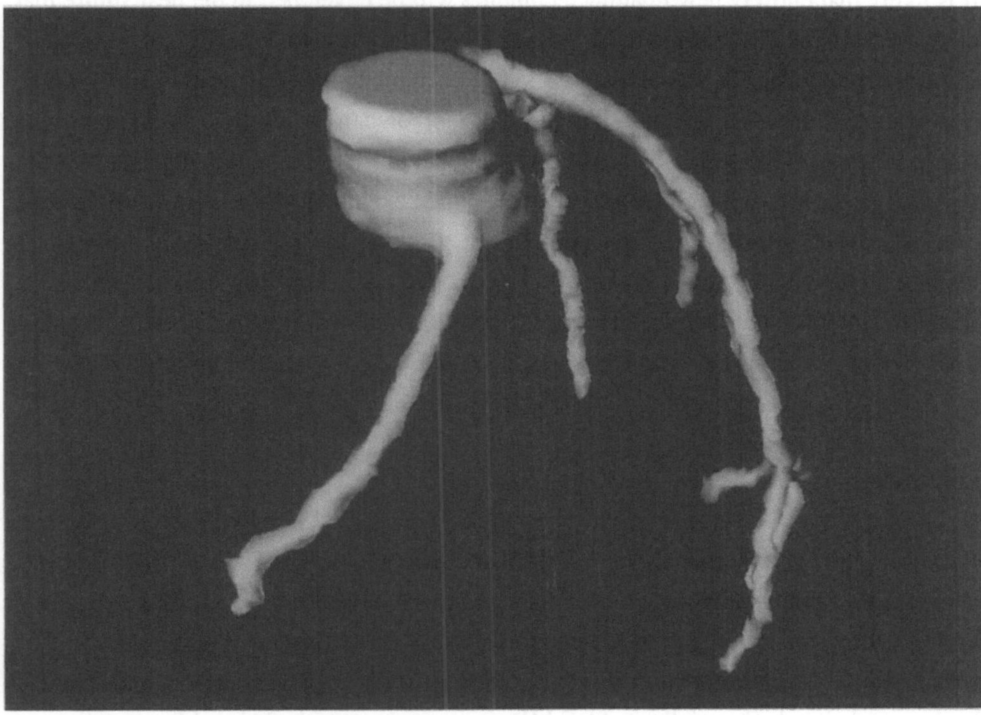

Fig. 1: Three-dimensional surface rendered display of a 3D EPI study of the proximal coronary tree obtained at 0.5 T. The 3D model is made up of 30-40 imaging slices that were obtained during a single breath-hold. The images were obtained with use of a dedicated cardiac surface coil and a fat suppression technique was used. Reproduced from ref. 15, with permission. Courtesy of Messrs. Jan Dam and Jan Vermeulen, Philips Medical Systems, Best, the Netherlands.

Most experience with coronary MR angiography has been gained with the fast gradient-echo techniques such as turbo-FLASH [13,14]. With this technique, the shortest imaging times for a single image with a 128 x 128 matrix is in the order of 300-350 msec. This is obviously too long to freeze the cardiac motion, and the acquisition is therefore "segmented" into multiple 100-msec-blocks of phase encoding steps which are obtained during consecutive heart beats. "Segmented turbo-FLASH" can acquire a 128 x 256 matrix single slice in 16 heartbeats [13]. By implementing stronger gradient coils in the MR magnet (which requires considerable engineering features to accomplish) the turbo-FLASH technique may be sped up somewhat further, up to the point where the major speed limiting factor relates to the application of the slice-selective excitation pulse which requires itself approximately 1 msec. This poses a speed limit of a 128 x 128 matrix image being acquired within approximately 130 msec.

It is likely that entirely new imaging techniques will be developed in the near future that are based on the EPI technique. Using specially designed coils, EPI can generate a 64x128 matrix image in 30 msec after a single excitation pulse (single shot EPI), which is sufficiently short to preclude blurring because of cardiac motion. A limitation of single shot EPI is the low SNR because of the relatively long echo time required for the read-out of the entire imaging plane after the single excitation pulse. As was discussed, long echo times result in more significant flow artifacts because of intravoxel dephasing. Hybrid techniques have been developed, whereby EPI is used to form an image with use of multiple (5-10) excitation pulses: multi-shot EPI. Recently, the first MR coronary angiograms made with multi-shot EPI have been published (Figure 1) [15].

Optimizing signal-to-noise-ratio

Because of the physiological constraints mentioned above, the SNR in MR coronary angiography is inherently low. Additional measures to enhance the SNR of the coronary arteries are therefore important as these may make the difference between success or failure of the MR examination. Of significant importance is adequate suppression of background signal. Especially in TOF MR angiography, residual signal from stationary fat may be an issue. Cancellation of the background signal depends on stationary spin saturation by the fast train of radiofrequency pulses. Fat (surrounding the coronary vessels) has short T1-relaxation time and maintains therefore some residual signal. This is the rationale for applying additional fat suppression with a fat-selective saturation pulse (Figure 2). Spins in fatty tissue resonate at a resonance frequency slightly different from that of spins in water molecules (chemical shift). A presaturation pulse at precisely the resonance frequency of fat is applied to the imaging volume. Consequently, the spins in fatty tissue are saturated and will not contribute any signal. The presaturation pulse will not influence the spins in water and will thus not interfere with MR angiography flow contrast.

Another measure to improve the SNR is by using intravascular MR contrast agents [16]. Contrast media such as the gadolinium-based compounds shorten the T1 relaxation time

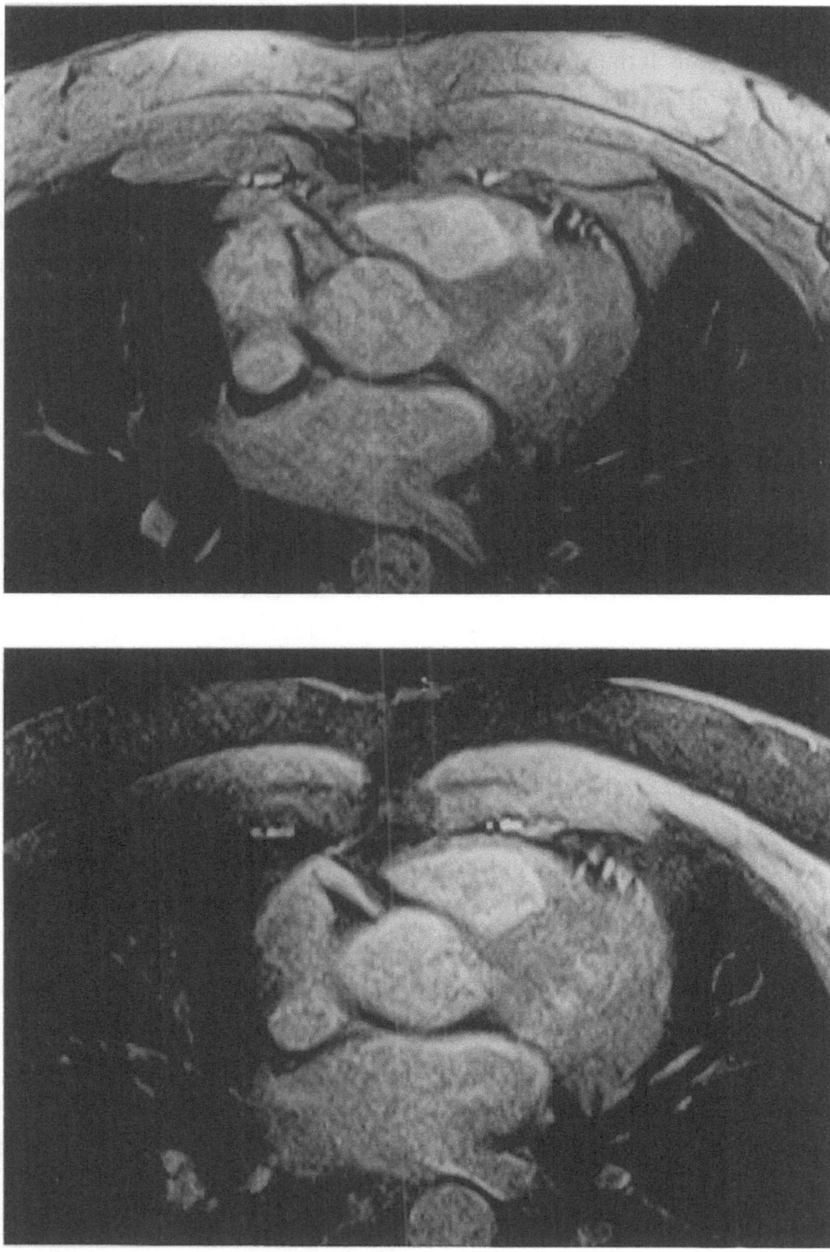

Fig. 2: The importance of fat suppression techniques in MR coronary angiography. Transverse MR images of the proximal right coronary artery. Without fat suppression (Fig. 2a) the coronary artery is not well visualized within the right atrioventricular groove. With fat suppression (Fig. 2b), on the other hand, the right coronary artery is clearly seen. Fast gradient echo MR coronary angiography performed at 1.5 T with use of a surface coil. Courtesy of Mr. Jan Dam, Philips Medical Systems, Best, the Netherlands.

of blood and hence increase the vascular signal relative to the surrounding tissue. Contrast agents appear to especially increase the image quality in diseased vessels with slow or poststenotic turbulent flow. They may be categorized according to their pharmacokinetic properties into extracellular agents (e.g., gadolinium-DTPA) and blood-pool agents (e.g., polymeric agents such as dextran-(gadolinium-DTPA)$_{15}$). The blood-pool agents have a longer plasma half-life than the extracellular agents, with only limited diffusion to the extracellular space, and this implies that the enhanced SNR is maintained for a longer period [17]. The blood-pool contrast media are currently investigational only. An additional two- to threefold SNR improvement is anticipated with the use of optimized phased-array surface coils replacing the conventional surface coils or the magnet system's body coil [18].

Initial results with MR coronary angiography

At this early stage in the development of the technique, the majority of studies have focussed on technical aspects of MR coronary angiography and the feasibility of applying the method in vivo. To date, only the proximal coronary tree and the relatively large size aortocoronary bypasses are visualized. Typically, one can see the proximal 8 cm of the right coronary artery, the proximal 5 cm of the left anterior descending artery and the proximal 1.5 cm of the circumflex artery [4,19]. The branches of the main coronary vessels are usually not reliably visualized (Figures 1, 3).

There are no firm data on the clinical utility of MR coronary angiography. Initial studies, all done with the turbo-FLASH sequence, suggest that the method needs to be further improved in order to become clinically useful. Manning et al. reported 90% sensitivity for detecting significant stenoses in 52 coronary arteries with moderately severe or severe disease on contrast angiography [13]. Other research groups, however, could not reproduce these good results. Duerinckx et al. obtained a sensitivity of 63% in 27 lesions [14], and Pennell et al. one of 65% in 23 stenoses [20]. Post and coworkers found a sensitivity of as low as 36% with a 2D technique (5 of 14 lesions detected) [21] and even of 0% in 17 lesions with a 3D technique [22].

Initial experience with MR flow mapping has focussed on the feasibility of in vivo flow measurements in the coronary arteries [23] and in (normal and stenosed) saphenous vein aortocoronary bypasses [24,25]. Under favorable circumstances it is possible to obtain good results in coronary arteries but the method is not yet robust. It is somewhat less of a problem to apply MR flow mapping to the larger caliber

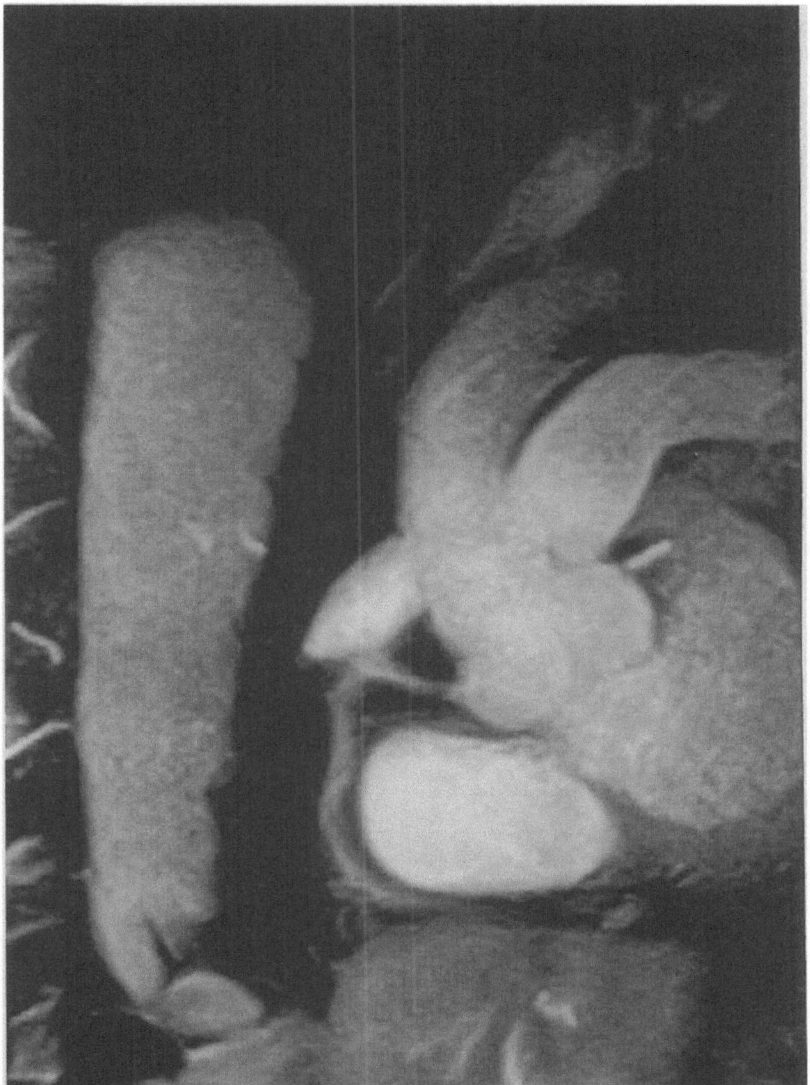

Fig. 3: MR coronary angiogram obtained during a single breath-hold. The image orientation is reminiscent of the right anterior oblique projection in conventional coronary angiography. Fast gradient echo MR angiographyt at 1.5 T, with use of fat suppression and a surface coil. Courtesy of Mr. Jan Dam, Philips Medical Systems, Best, the Netherlands.

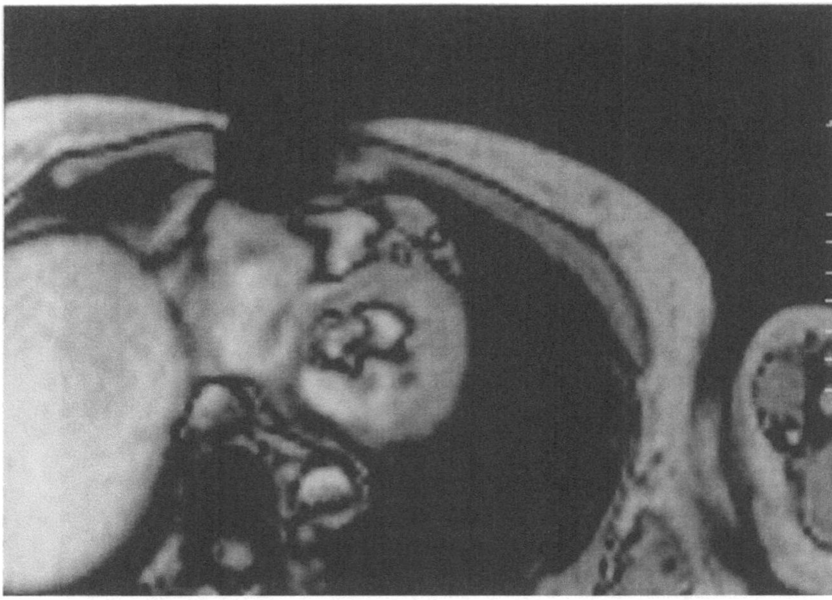

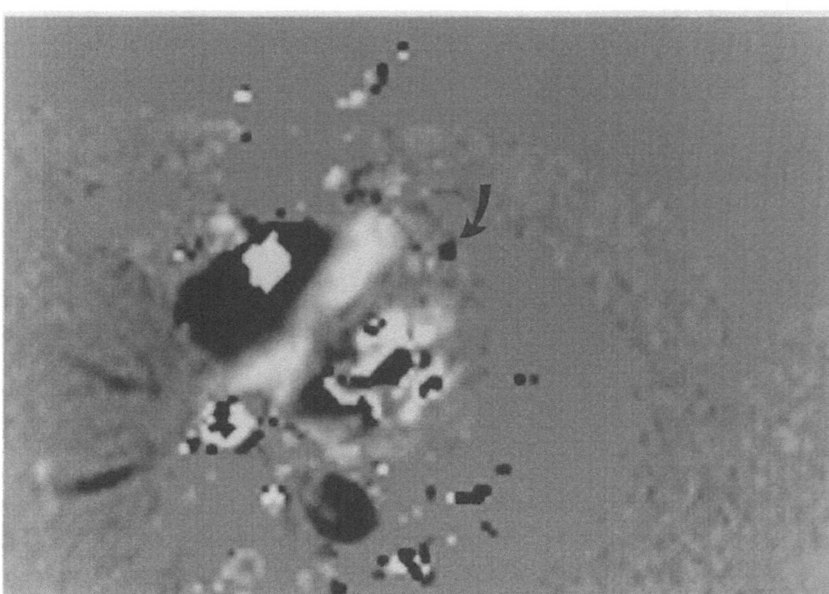

Fig. 4: MR images of a saphenous vein bypass graft to the left anterior descending artery performed at 0.5 T with a body coil. The modulus image (Fig. 4a) and the corresponding phase encoded velocity image from MRI flow mapping (Fig. 4b) both show a flow signal indicating graft patency.

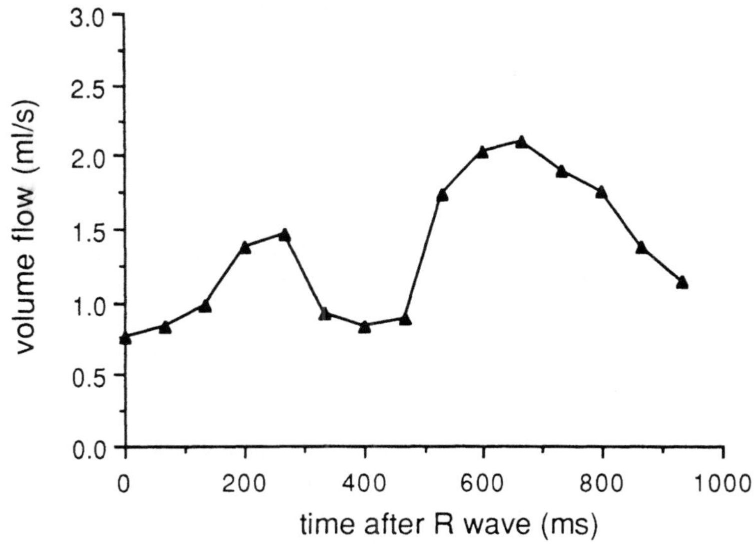

The flow curve has a biphasic profile (Fig. 4c); the graft flow volume is 78 ml/min. Reproduced from ref.25, with permission.

venous bypasses (Figure 4). It is important, however convincing the initial results may seem, that one keeps in mind that the method is only validated with regard to its use in large size vessels such as the aorta. There are no published studies which have firmly validated the flow measurements in the small caliber coronary arteries.

Conclusion

Currently, MR coronary angiography should be regarded as an experimental method only. The angiographic images are clearly inferior to conventional X-ray coronary angiography in terms of spatial and time resolution. The measurements of volume flow appear to be promising but are not yet validated. This, however, may change in the near future with further technical improvements. Dedicated cardiac MR hardware (gradient coils for EPI, phased array coils), MR software (imaging sequences, fat suppression) and use of MR contrast agents will improve the results of coronary MR angiography. A drawback of MR coronary angiography at the present time is the high cost of this dedicated equipment. Despite its current limitations, coronary MR angiography is a promising technique which, as a noninvasive examination, may be performed on an outpatient basis. Even if the MR angiography evaluation would be restricted to the proximal portions of the coronary arteries, it may well turn out to be a cost-effective method for screening patients with chronic angina.

References

1. White HD, Cross DB, Elliott JM, Norris RM, Yee TW. Long-term prognostic importance of patency of the infarct-related coronary artery after thrombolytic therapy for acute myocardial infarction. Circulation 1994;89:61-7.
2. Siebert JE, Pernicone JR, Potchen EJ. Physical principles and application of magnetic resonance angiography. Semin Ultrasound CT MRI 1992;13:227-45.
3. Edelman RR. MR angiography: present and future. AJR AM J Roentgenol 1993;161:1-11.
4. Manning WJ, Li W, Boyle NG, Edelman RR. Fat-suppressed breath-hold magnetic resonance coronary angiography. Circulation 1993;87:94-104.
5. Li D, Paschal CB, Haacke EM, Adler LP. Coronary arteries: three-dimensional MR imaging with fat saturation and magnetization transfer contrast. Radiology 1993;187:401-6.
6. Wang S, Hu B, Macovski A, Nishimura D. Coronary angiography using fast selective inversion recovery. Magn Reson Med 1991;18:417-23.
7. Edelman RR, Siewert B, Adamis M, Gaa J, Laub G, Wielopolski P. Signal targeting with alternating radiofrequency (STAR) sequences: application to MR angiography. Magn Reson Med 1994;31:233-8.
8. Laub G. Displays for MR angiography. Magn Reson Med 1990;14:222-9.
9. Anderson CM, Saloner D, Shapeero LG, Lee RE. Artifacts in maximum-intensity-projection displays of MR angiograms. AJR AM J Roentgenol 1990;154:623-9.
10. Keegan J, Firmin P, Gatehouse D, Longmore DB. The application of breath hold phase velocity mapping techniques to the measurements of coronal artery blood flow velocity: phantom data and initial in vivo results. Magn Reson Med 1994;31:526-36.
11. Haacke EM, Tkach JA. Fast MR imaging: techniques and clinical applications. AJR Roentgenol 1990;155:951-64.
12. Wehrli FW. Fast-scan magnetic resonance: principles and applications. Magn Reson Q 1990; 6:165-236.
13. Manning WJ, Li W, Edelman RR. A preliminary report comparing magnetic resonance coronary imaging angiography with conventional angiography. N Engl J Med 1993; 328:828-32.
14. Duerinckx AJ, Urman M. Two-dimensional coronary MR angiography: analysis of initial clinical results. Radiology 1994; 193:731-8.
15. Börnert P, Jensen D. Coronary artery imaging at 0.5 T using echo planar imaging. Proc Soc Magn Reson 1994;2:372.
16. Duerinckx AJ, Urman M, Sinha U, Atkinson D, Simonetti O. Evaluation of gadolinium-enhanced MR coronary angiography [abstract]. Radiology 1993;189 (Suppl P:278.
17. Brasch RC, Weissleder R. Trends and new developments in MRI contrast enhancement. In: Brasch RC, editor. MRI contrast enhancement in the central nervous system: a case study approach. New York: Raven Press, 1993:301-26.

18. Chien D, Anderson C. Breathhold magnetic resonance angiography of coronary arteries using a circularly polarized phased array system. Proc Soc Magn Reson 1994;2:502.
19. Pennell DJ, Keegan J, Firmin DN, Gatehouse PD, Underwood SR, Longmore DB. Magnetic resonance imaging of coronary arteries: technique and preliminary results. Br Heart J 1993; 70:315-26.
20. Pennell DJ, Bogren HG, Keegan J, Firmin DW, Underwood SR. Coronary artery stenosis: assessment by magnetic resonance imaging [abstract]. In: Proceedings of the 11th annual scientific meeting of the European Society for Magnetic Resonance in Medicine and Biology, 1994. Vienna:S.N., 1994:401.
21. Post JC, Van Rossum AC, Hofman MBM, Valk J, Visser CA. Current limitations of two dimensional breath hold MR angiography in coronary artery disease. Proc Soc Magn Reson 1994;2:509.
22. Post JC, Van Rossum AC, Hofman MBM, Valk J, Visser CA. Respiratory-gated three dimensional MR angiography of coronary arteries and comparison with X-ray contrast angiography [abstract]. Proceedings of the Society of Magnetic Resonance. 2nd meeting, August 1994, San Francisco:509.
23. Edelman RR, Manning WJ, Gervino E, Li W. Flow velocity quantification in human coronary arteries with fast, breath-hold MR angiography. J Magn Reson Imaging 1993; 3:699-703.
24. Galjee MA, Van Rossum AC, Doesburg T, Visser CA. Non-invasive assessment of coronary artery graft patency and flow rate by magnetic resonance imaging [abstract]. J Am Coll Cardiol 1994;(Special issue):297A.
25. Hoogendoorn LI, Pattynama PMT, Buis B, Van der Geest RJ, Van der Wall EE, De Roos A. Noninvasive evaluation of aortocoronary bypass grafts with magnetic resonance flow mapping. Am J Cardiol. In Press.

Noninvasive imaging of coronary artery anomalies

Present angiographic criteria and role of additional techniques, especially fast gradient echo magnetic resonance imaging

H.W. Vliegen[*], J. Doornbos[**], J.W. Jukema[*], M.A. Bekedam[*], A. de Roos[**] and E.E. van der Wall[*]

[*] *Department of Cardiology, University Hospital Leiden, the Netherlands*

[**] *Department of Diagnostic Radiology, University Hospital Leiden, the Netherlands*

Summary

Determination of the course of an aberrant coronary artery using coronary arteriography is often difficult. Fast gradient echo magnetic resonance (MR) angiography, however, can be a useful additional technique in case coronary arteriography is inconclusive. In this chapter, the different types of coronary artery anomalies are reviewed, arteriographic criteria are discussed, the technique of fast gradient echo MR angiography is described, results with this technique are shown and the various other additional diagnostic techniques are discussed.

Fast gradient echo magnetic resonance angiography appears to be a useful additional technique to coronary arteriography for the analysis of the true course of aberrant coronary arteries.

Introduction

The unsuspected anomalous origin of coronary arteries is an important potential problem in any catheterization laboratory. The natural history and treatment of these arteries is more dependent on the initial course of the anomalous vessel rather than its site of origin. The angiographer has the critical responsibility of accurately defining the origin and course, as well as the degree of atherosclerosis in such vessels.

By probing the 3 coronary cusps with standard catheters in the left anterior oblique view the origin of anomalous coronary arteries is usually easy to identify. However, since angiography only provides a 2-dimensional view of a complex 3-dimensional

E. E. van der Wall et al. (eds.), Advances in Imaging Techniques in Ischemic Heart Disease 47–58.

structure it is often difficult, even for experienced angiographers to delineate the proximal course of the anomalous vessels. In a high percentage of cases, the anatomy of the coronary arteries is not established correctly. Ishikawa et al. reevaluated 24 published cases in which the left main coronary artery originated anomalously from the right anterior aortic sinus or proximal right coronary artery [1]. They found misdiagnosis to be surprisingly common, occurring in up to 50% of cases. Especially a septal course was often misdiagnosed as being interarterial. This stresses the need for additional techniques for the analysis of the true course of aberrant coronary arteries.

The incidence of coronary anomalies

Important anatomical variations in origin and distribution of coronary arteries are diagnosed in approximately 1% of patients undergoing coronary arteriography [2]. About 80% of these anomalies are benign and do not cause signs or symptoms. They are incidental findings at the moment of catheterization, or are discovered during autopsy. Approximately 20% of these anomalies are potentially malignant as they may cause myocardial ischemia resulting in angina pectoris, myocardial infarction, syncope, arrhythmias, heart failure, and sudden death [2]. Therefore, it is of great importance to distinguish the benign from the malignant anomalies. Table 1 shows the different coronary anomalies, with their incidence and their relative percentage based on a study including 126,595 patients [2]. It should be noted that the exact incidence of coronary anomalies in a normal population is unknown, but evidently lower than the 1% mentioned in the study of Yamanaka and Hobbs [2], since all 126,595 patients in that study must have had a reason to undergo coronary arteriography. Such a reason may have been ischemia related cardiac complaints resulting from the aberrant coronary artery.

The left main originating from the contralateral sinus

When the left main coronary artery arises anomalously from the right sinus Valsalvae or the proximal right coronary artery, its course can be divided into 4 anatomical subtypes. These four types are: 1) an interarterial course, between aorta and pulmonary artery (malignant); 2) a septal course, between aorta and right ventricular outflow tract (benign); 3) a retro aortic course (benign); and 4) a course anterior to the arteria pulmonalis (benign). The septal type is the most common and is considered relatively harmless. The interarterial type is the dangerous anomaly. Symptoms, like sudden death, occur mainly in young individuals during physical exercise. It has been postulated that exercise results in the expansion of the aorta, which may occlude acutely the angulated slit-like orifice of the left main artery [2].

When the left main coronary artery arises anomalously from the right sinus Valsalvae, or from the proximal right coronary artery, cine-angiography may reveal the four following possibilities: 1) a cranial posterior loop of the anomalous left main coronary artery indicating an interarterial course, 2) a caudal anterior loop indicating a septal course, 3) a caudal posterior loop indicating a retro-aortic course, and 4) a cranial anterior loop indicating a course anterior to the arteria pulmonalis [1].

An additional method for rapid identification of the course of anomalous coronary arteries is the 'dot and eye' method [3] (Table 2). Using this method, the four possibilities are differentiated as follows:

Interarterial course: the left main coronary artery courses between the aorta and pulmonary artery to its normal position on the anterior surface of the heart. It divides into the left anterior descending and circumflex coronary arteries at the point where it normally does and thus gives rise to a left anterior descending (RDA) and circumflex (CX) coronary arteries of normal length and course. During right anterior oblique (RAO) ventriculography the left main coronary artery will appear as a radiopaque 'dot' anterior to the aorta.

Septal course: the left main coronary artery runs an intramuscular course through the ventricular septum along the floor of the right ventricular outflow tract. It then surfaces in the midseptum at which point it branches into the left anterior descending and the left circumflex coronary arteries. Because the artery divides in the midseptum, the initial portion of the circumflex courses toward the aorta (the normal position of the proximal left anterior descending artery (RDA)) and the RDA is thus relatively short. During 30 degree right anterior oblique coronary arteriography, the left main coronary artery and the initial portion of the circumflex artery will form an ellipse to the left of the aorta similar to an 'eye' with the left main coronary artery forming the inferior portion and the circumflex forming the superior portion. An additional clue to the septal course is the presence of septal perforator branches arising from the left main coronary artery.

Retroaortic course: The left main coronary artery passes posteriorly around the aortic root to its normal position on the anterior surface of the heart. It divides into the left anterior descending and circumflex arteries at the point where it normally does and thus gives rise to a RDA and CX of normal length and course. During 30 degree right anterior oblique ventriculography the left main will appear as a radiopaque 'dot', posterior to the aorta.

Table 1: The incidence of isolated coronary artery anomalies from a total of 126,595 patients (from Yamanaka and Hobbs [2]).

Anomalies	Incidence (%)	% of total
Benign		
Separate origin of LAD and CX in LSV	0.41	30.4
CX from RSV or RCA with retroaortic course	0.37	27.7
Coronary artery from PSV		
LM from PSV	0.0008	0.06
RCA from PSV	0.003	0.24
Anomalous origin from ascending aorta above SV		
LM from aorta	0.013	0.95
RCA from aorta	0.15	11.2
Absent CX ("super-dominant RCA")	0.003	0.24
Intercoronary communication	0.002	0.18
Small coronary artery fistulae	0.12	9.7
Total	1.07	80.6
Potentially serious		
Coronary artery from pulmonary artery		
LM from PA	0.008	0.59
LAD from PA	0.0008	0.06
RCA from PA	0.002	0.12
CX from PA	not mentioned	
Coronary artery from opposite aortic sinus		
LM from RSV	0.017	1.3
LAD from RSV	0.03	2.3
RCA from LSV	0.107	8.1
CX from RSV (frontal to aorta)	not mentioned	
Single coronary artery		
originating from RSV	0.020	1.5
originating from LSV	0.025	1.9
Multiple or large sized fistulae	0.05	3.7
Total	0.26	19.4

Abbreviations:

CX, circumflex artery; LAD, left anterior descending artery; LM, left main; LSV, left sinus of Valsalva; PA, pulmonary artery; PSV, posterior sinus of Valsalva; RCA, right coronary artery; RSV, right sinus of Valsalva; SV, sinus Valsalvae.

Table 2: Radiographic appearance of anomalous origin of the left main coronary artery from the right sinus of Valsalva.

	RAO Arteriography or Ventriculography			
Course of Anomalous LM	Dot	Eye	LAD length	Septals from LM
Interarterial	+ anterior	-	normal	no
Septal	-	+ upper CX lower LM	short	yes
Retroaortic	+ posterior	-	normal	no
Anterior	-	+ lower CX	short	no

Anterior free wall course: The left main coronary artery crosses the anterior free wall of the right ventricle (the initial course is similar to the course of the normal conus branch) and then divides at the midseptum into the RDA and circumflex. Because the artery divides at the midseptum, the initial portion of the circumflex artery courses toward the aorta (the normal position of the proximal RDA) and the RDA is relatively short. During right anterior oblique coronary arteriography the left main coronary artery and the initial portion of the circumflex artery will form an ellipse ('eye') to the left of the aorta, with the left main coronary artery forming the superior portion and the circumflex artery forming the inferior portion. The septal and anterior course are distinguished by whether the left main coronary artery forms the lower or the upper portion of the ellipse, respectively.

Although these angiographic criteria are very useful, considerable doubt about the true course of the anomaly may arise if the required projections are missing, or the interpreter is unaware of the exact projections. In these cases, additional techniques are needed.

Fast gradient echo MR angiography

Technique

Patients were examined in prone position with a Philips Gyroscan 1.5 Tesla MR-scanner. Images were acquired using a circular surface coil (17 cm diameter) positioned at the level of the aortic root. Gradient echo scout views were obtained in the coronal, sagittal and transverse plane, comprising the left ventricle and the aortic root. These surveys are used to define the oblique transverse and oblique sagittal sections for gradient echo MR angiography. Experience is required to locate the optimal views. The images were obtained using a segmented fast gradient echo sequence with a repetition time of 15 ms, an echo time of 6 ms, and a pulse angle of 50 degrees. Slice thickness is 4 mm, field of view 25 cm x 17.5 cm. The ECG-triggered end-diastolic data acquisition is segmented over 16 heart beats during breath hold. Acquisition time is therefore dependent on the heart rate, e.g. 18 s per image at a cardiac frequency of 55 beats per minute. The acquired data matrix is 256 x 112, displayed as a 256 x 180 pixel image. Epicardial fat signal is suppressed using a spectrally selective radio frequency prepulse.

Fast gradient echo MR angiography of a healthy volunteer

Figure 1 shows a fast gradient echo MR angiography of a healthy volunteer. While interpreting an MR angiographic image, one has to realize that it concerns a caudal view. Therefore the right coronary artery is seen on the left side on the image and the left main stem is projected at the right side of the aorta. The anterior chest wall of the patient is seen at the top of the image.
The image of the healthy volunteer clearly displays the origin of the left main stem from the left sinus Valsalvae, and the origin of the right coronary artery from the right sinus Valsalvae. The illustration clearly displays the branching of the left main stem into the left anterior descending artery (LAD) and the circumflex artery (CX).

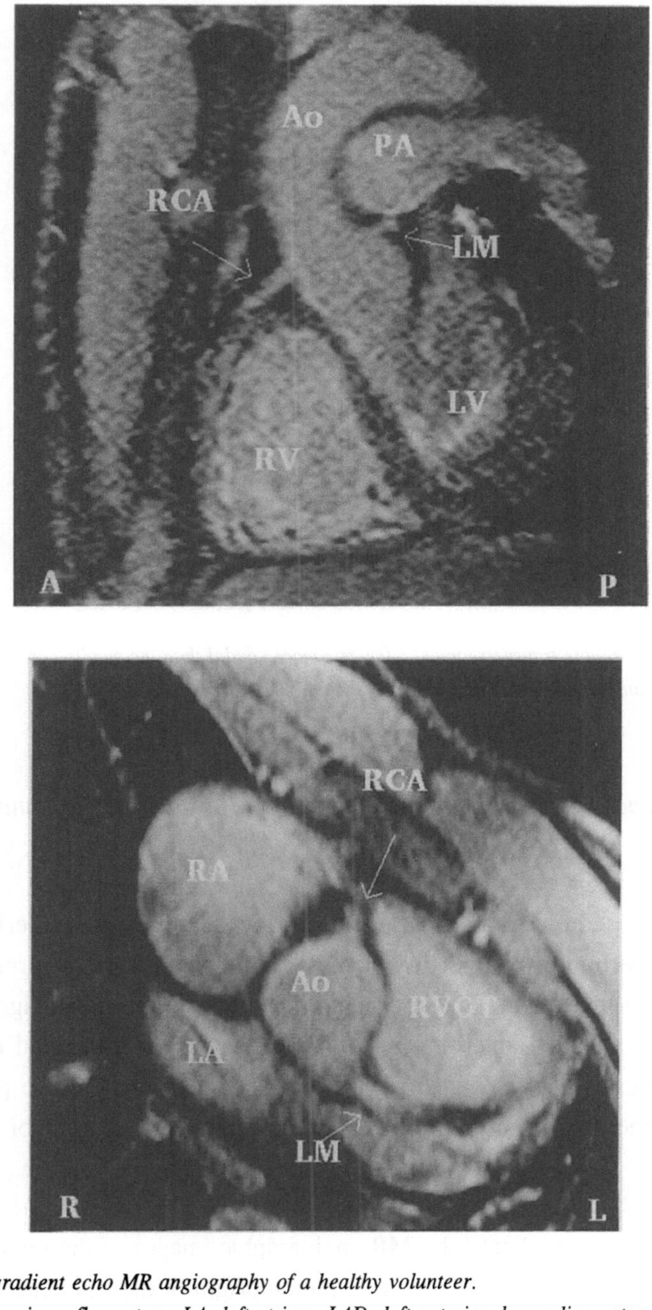

Fig. 1: Fast gradient echo MR angiography of a healthy volunteer.
Ao, aorta; Cx, circumflex artery; LA, left atrium; LAD, left anterior descending artery; LM, left main; LV, left ventricle; PA, pulmonary artery; RA, right atrium; RCA, right coronary artery; RV, right ventricle; RVOT, right ventricular outflow tract.
Upper panel (Fig. 1a). Oblique sagittal view. Note the left main and right coronary artery originating from the aorta. Middle panel (Fig.1b). Oblique transverse view. Left main and right coronary artery originate from the aorta.

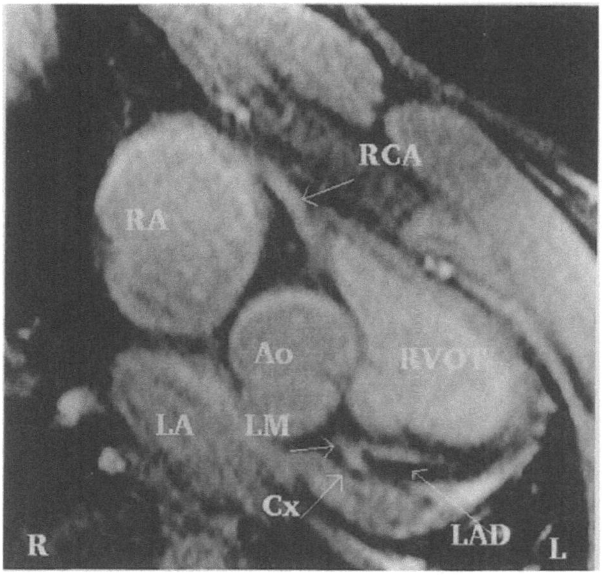

Lower panel (Fig. 1c). Oblique transverse view, a few mm more caudal than the middle panel. The left main branches into the left anterior descending artery and the left circumflex.

Example of diagnosing a coronary anomaly by MR angiography and coronary arteriography

Figure 2 displays a coronary arteriogram of a patient in the right anterior oblique projection after injection of contrast in a common ostium of the right coronary artery and an aberrant left main stem. The left main stem originates from the right coronary artery and follows a caudal anterior course. This suggests an intraseptal course [3]. Such a caudal anterior course is also referred to as a "hammock". The presence of septal branches emerging from the left main is another indication in favor of a septal course [3].

Figure 3 shows the fast gradient echo MR angiographic images of the same patient as shown in Figure 2. In the upper image the common origin of the right coronary artery and the left main is visualized. On the more caudal images the course through the interventricular septum can be followed.

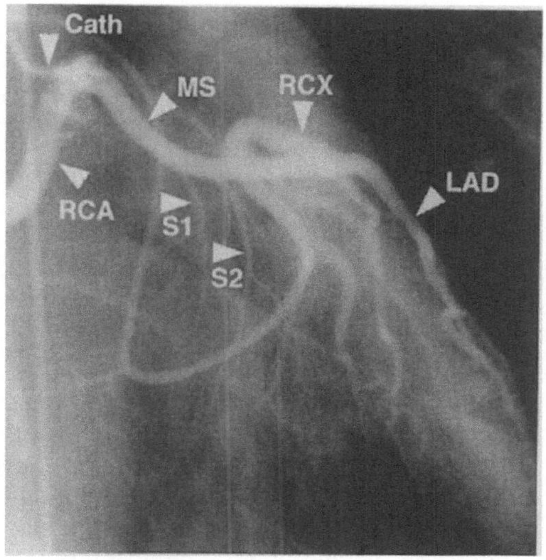

Fig. 2: Coronary arteriogram (right anterior oblique view) of a patient with a main stem originating from the right coronary artery and running through the interventricular septum. The catheter (Cath) is situated in the common ostium. From here the right coronary artery (RCA) and the left main stem (MS) originate. The main stem has a caudal and frontal course and septal branches (S1 en S2) arise from it. This favors a septal course. Afterwards the main stem branches in the left circumflex (CX) and left anterior descending artery (LAD).

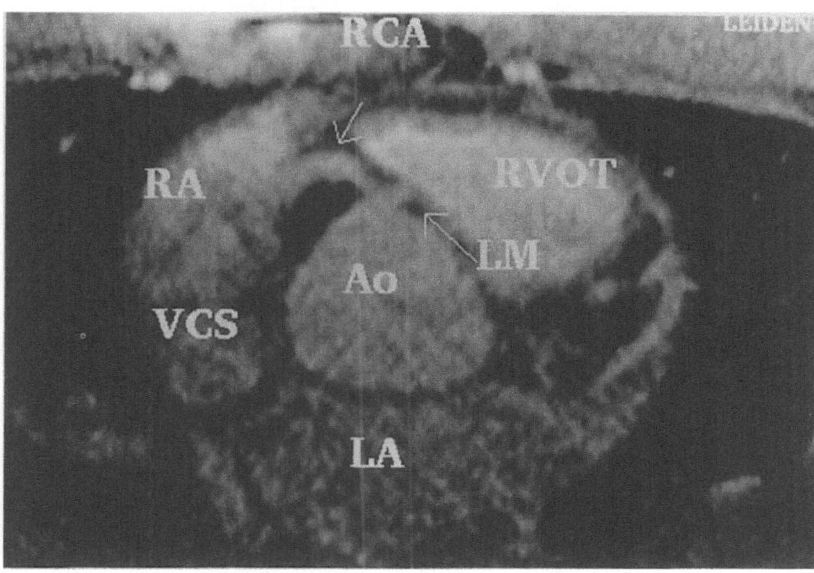

Fig. 3: Fast gradient echo MR angiography of the same patient as in Figure 2.
Upper panel (Fig. 3a). Oblique transverse view. Note the left main originating from the right coronary artery. Ao, aorta; IVS, interventricular septum; LA, left atrium; LM, left main; RA, right atrium; RCA, right coronary artery; RV, right ventricle; RVOT, right ventricular outflow tract.

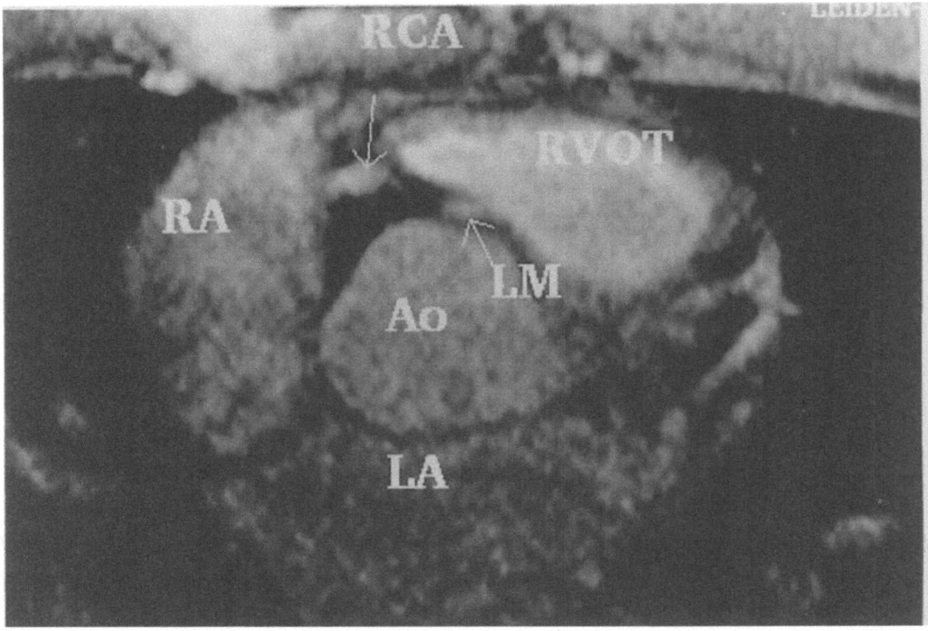

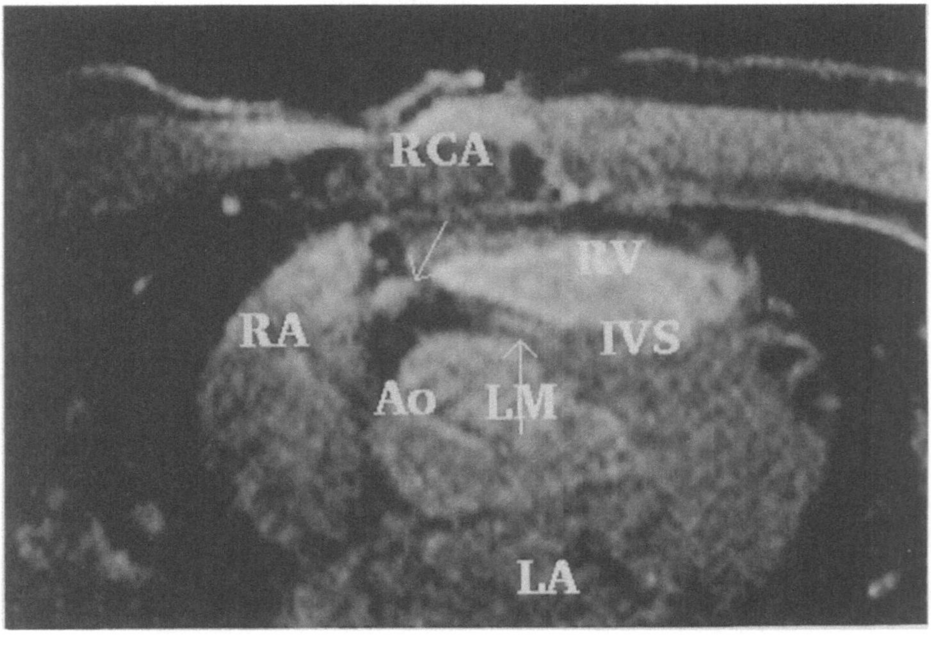

Middle panel (Fig. 3b). Oblique transverse view, a few mm more caudal than the upper panel. The left main runs between aorta and right ventricular outflow tract.
Lower panel (Fig. 3c). Oblique transverse view, a few mm more caudal than the middle panel. Note the left main (LM) runs through the interventricular septum (IVS).

Additional techniques

Both transesophageal echocardiography [4] and spin echo MR imaging [5] have been reported to be useful for analyzing the course of aberrant coronary arteries. Fernandes et al. investigated the aberrant coronary arteries of nine patients with transesophageal echocardiography using color Doppler. The abnormal orifice of the coronary arteries could be determined in all nine patients using this technique. In four patients in which the left main coronary originated from the right sinus Valsalvae, echocardiography displayed more insight in the followed course related to the aorta and the arteria pulmonalis than coronary arteriography. A disadvantage of transesophageal echocardiography is its semi-invasive character. Besides, the echocardiographic images displayed only a moderate contrast to noise ratio which made these difficult to interpret. Doorey et al. [5] described five patients with aberrant coronary arteries who could not be properly diagnosed with coronary arteriography in which spin-echo MR was used to diagnose the precise course of the aberrant coronary artery. It concerned three patients with an aberrant right coronary artery and two patients with an aberrant left coronary artery.

Gradient echo magnetic resonance angiography, is a relatively new MR imaging technique. The application of gradient echo MR angiography to visualize coronary arteries has recently been described by Manning and Edelman [6].

An important advantage of MR imaging compared to coronary arteriography is the visualization of both the artery and its surrounding anatomic structures. A disadvantage of MR imaging is the difficulty to follow the coronary arteries during a long course in the same scan plane, as a result of their curved anatomy. An advantage of coronary arteriography is the possibility of imaging the complete coronary artery. A disadvantage is that coronary arteriography only provides a 2-dimensional view of the complex 3-dimensional structure and that no information is obtained about the surrounding structures.

Specific advantages of MR imaging as compared to transesophageal echocardiography are the non-invasive character and the relatively high spatial resolution. An advantage of fast gradient echo MR angiography as compared to spin echo MR is the possibility of the patient to hold his breath during the image acquisition, thereby improving image quality. This causes a minimum of breathing artifacts and improves spatial resolution. MR imaging can be performed on an out-patient base without evident risks. The majority of the patients is accessible to investigation with MR. Contraindications of MR imaging are metal objects, such as pacemakers, cochlear implants, metal vessel clips because of aneurysms, and vessel stents in the first six weeks after implantation.

Pregnancy during the first three months is considered a relative contraindication. Claustrophobia prohibits the MR investigation in 2-5% of patients.

Conclusion

Fast gradient echo magnetic resonance angiography appears to be a useful additional technique to coronary arteriography for the analysis of the true course of aberrant coronary arteries in case coronary arteriography is inconclusive.

An important advantage of fast gradient echo MR angiography compared to coronary arteriography is the visualization of both the artery and its surrounding tissue. Fast gradient echo MR angiography is a non-invasive technique that provides excellent spatial resolution.

References

1. Ishikawa T. Brandt P. Anomalous origin of the left main coronary artery from the right anterior aortic sinus: angiographic definition of anomalous course. Am J Cardiol 1985;55:770-6.
2. Yamanaka O, Hobbs RE. Coronary artery anomalies in 126,595 patients undergoing coronary arteriography. Cathet Cardiovasc Diagn 1990;21:28-40.
3. Serota H, Barth CW, Seuc CA, Vandormael M, Aguirre F, Kern M. Rapid identification of the course of anomalous coronary arteries in adults: the "dot" and "eye" method. Am J Cardiol 1990;65:891-898.
4. Fernandes F, Alam M, Smith S, Khaja F. The role of transesophageal echocardiography in identifying anomalous coronary arteries. Circulation 1993;88:2532-40.
5. Doorey AJ, Wills JS, Blasetto J, Goldenberg EM. Usefulness of magnetic resonance imaging for diagnosing an anomalous coronary artery coursing between aorta and pulmonary trunk. Am J Cardiol 1994;74:198-199.
6. Manning WJ, Edelman RR: Magnetic resonance coronary angiography [Review]. Magn Reson Q 1993;9:131-51.

Left ventricular function by stress MR imaging

Animal studies using dobutamine

J. Baan* **and P.M.T. Pattynama****

**Department of Cardiology, **Department of Diagnostic Radiology and Nucleair Medicine, Leiden University Hospital, the Netherlands*

Summary

The study describes the application of end-systolic pressure-volume relations (ESPVR) to assess cardiac contractility and pump function and how these quantities change with stress. Pressure-volume loops were constructed in ten anesthetized pigs, using both MRI and the conductance catheter to obtain left ventricular volume, combined with a special micromanometer-tip catheter for pressure measurement. The loops were obtained both during normal and reduced hemodynamic loading conditions, the latter acquired bij nitroprusside. Stress conditions were induced by dobutamine at an infusion rate of 10 μg/kg/min.

The ESPVR showed a parallel leftward shift (decreasing volume intercept) with dobutamine, indicating increased contractile state. The leftward shift was similar for the two methods: 6.9 ml for MRI and 7.4 ml for the conductance catheter method on the average. The slope of the ESPVR did not change significantly for either method. This finding is in agreement with results obtained by other investigators.

It is concluded that, just as had been shown previously for the conductance method, pressure-volume loops and -relations may be obtained reliably using MRI for left ventricular volume measurement. This is promising for future applications of MRI to assess pump function during dobutamine-induced stress in patients diagnosed for left ventricular dysfunction.

E. E. van der Wall et al. (eds.), Advances in Imaging Techniques in Ischemic Heart Disease 59–70.

Introduction

To assess pump function and contractility of the left ventricle, measurement of volume as a phasic signal during the cardiac cycle in addition to LV pressure is required. Such a measurement, namely, enables one to construct pressure-volume loops, from which, after a loading intervention, essentially all of the following information can be derived:
1) diastolic pressure-volume relation, from which diastolic LV distensibility or stiffness constant may be computed [1];
2) end-systolic pressure-volume relation (ESPVR), the slope (E_{es}) and volume intercept (V_d) which provide information on the contractile state of the LV [2,3];
3) the maximal derivative of pressure (dP/dt_{max}) as a function of end-diastolic volume (EDV) [4];
4) stroke work as a function of EDV: preload-recruitable stroke work [5]. The slopes of the latter two relationships also reflect contractility in a way much less dependent on changes in preload (EDV) and afterload (aortic pressure or impedance) than traditionally used indices such as ejection fraction, velocity of circumferential fiber shortening, v_{cf}, or dP/dt_{max}.
We have shown previously that P-V loops in the intact animal preparation as well as in man may be obtained using the conductance catheter developed in our laboratory to measure LV volume along with pressure [6]. The method has been used successfully to assess changes in contractile performance using dobutamine, both in animals and man [7,8,9,10]. The conductance catheter, however, requires calibration in order to obtain volume in an absolute sense, certainly in patients with enlarged ventricles such as present in heart failure [11,12]. The present study addresses the question whether P-V loops may be obtained using magnetic resonance imaging (MRI) using a vasodilator to obtain preload and afterload reduction, and dobutamine to change contractility. In order to compare the changes in the ESPVR (constructed by load changes) before and after dobutamine, the studies were performed sequentially in the same animal using the conductance catheter as well as MRI.

Methods and materials

Studies were performed in ten female piglets with body mass 25-33 kg (mean 27.5 kg). After intramuscular injection of atropine (0.05 mg/kg) the animals were anesthetized with intraperitoneal metomidate (Hypnodil, 20 mg/kg) and intravenous azaperon (Stresnil, 2 mg/kg). They were intubated and anesthesia was maintained by inhalation of 0.5% isoflurane supplemented with intravenous boluses of azaperon (1 mg/kg every

90 min) and 100 mg boluses of metomidate whenever required. Physical signs, blood pressure and ECG were used to monitor anesthesia and hemodynamic stability. Ventilation was monitored by capnography and sodium bicarbonate was administered to maintain normal pH. To block compensatory sympathetic and parasympathetic reflexes, 4 mg metoprolol (Selokene) and 1 mg atropine were administered intravenously every 30 min of the experiment.

After sheaths were inserted into the right jugular vein and both carotid arteries, all catheters were introduced under fluoroscopic control. A special 5F catheter-tip micromanometer (model SPC-350MR, Millar, Houston, TX) was positioned in the LV cavity. Because of its special construction in brass this manometer produces only small artifacts caused by MR, and allows recording of high-fidelity pressures during the studies without disturbing endocardial borders in the MR images [13]. The manometer catheter was calibrated before the data acquisition and calibration was checked after completion of the experiment. Before performing the imaging studies, a 7F, 12-electrode conductance catheter (Webster Labs, Baldwin Park, CA), with electrode spacing to match the length (6-7 cm) of the LV, was placed along the LV long axis with its tip in the apex, through the right carotid artery. For volume calibration purposes, a Berman balloon-flotation catheter (Arrow Int., Reading, PA) was positioned in the pulmonary artery, approached via the jugular vein. This catheter was used for injection of a small bolus of hypertonic saline (see below). The Berman and the conductance catheter were removed before the start of the imaging studies, the latter because the presence of the stainless-steel ring-shaped electrodes distorts the MR images.

Volume measurement by MRI and conductance catheter

Multisection gradient echo (cine) MR imaging was performed at 1.5 Tesla (Gyroscan, Philips Medical Systems, Best, Netherlands) using a 30^0 flip angle. Because ECG triggering failed in a pilot experiment, image acquisition was triggered using the peak positive dP/dt signal, which proved satisfactory in all studies [14,15]. Echo time was 13 ms and repetition time was equal to the duration of the cardiac cycle. MRI data were acquired by a 128x128 matrix with a field view of 30x30 cm^2, and a 256x256 matrix-display image was formed. A scout image was obtained in the sagittal plane to identify the position of the apex and the ascending aorta and to measure the angulation of the LV long axis. As the porcine heart is positioned in the midline, pointing anterocaudally, short axis imaging planes could be constructed using the scout view by electronically rotating the transverse plane around the left-to-right axis. The heart was imaged from apex to base with 7 contiguous imaging sections of 10 mm thickness. Each ventricular section level was imaged separately to achieve a time resolution of 26-28 ms, which is equivalent to achieve a time resolution of 36-38 frames per s, or 16-27 time frames per cardiac cycle, depending on heart rate. The first time frame was timed at 8 ms after the trigger pulse. All electronic equipment was positioned outside the magnetic field at a distance of at least 10 m from the MR magnet, and the infusion pumps were positioned approximately 3 m from the magnet.

To avoid observer bias, imaging runs were assigned a random number at the time of data acquisition. The observer was thus unaware of the identity of the animal, its hemodynamic condition and contractile state. Image analysis was performed using standardized criteria [16], modified to account for the smaller heart size in piglets as compared to the human heart. For analysis the images were displayed on a computer monitor in a movie-loop mode. In all time frames, endocardial borders were outlined manually with a trackball cursor and the enclosed surface areas were measured by computer. The 7 surface areas were summed, multiplied by section thickness to obtain ventricular volume. The 16-27 volume values obtained per cardiac cycle were plotted versus time. Subsequently, the curves were interpolated using a cubic-spline fitting algorithm [17] to obtain volume data at the same time resolution as the pressure data (5 ms sample period). The volume curves thus obtained were combined with the pressure curves to construct pressure-volume loops (Figure 1).

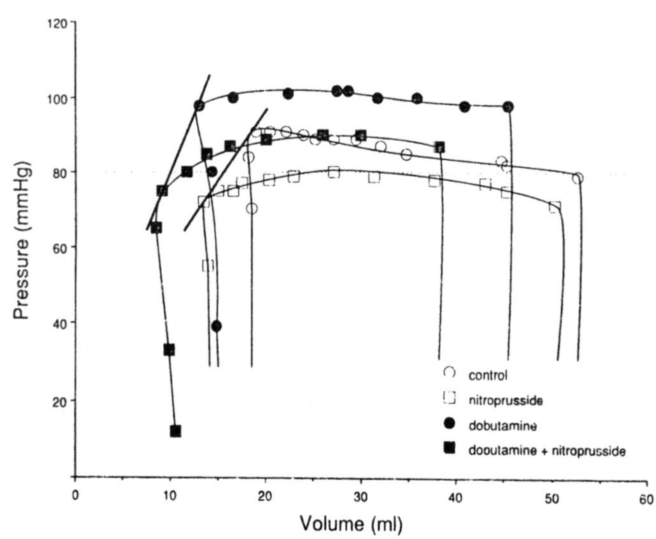

Fig. 1: Pressure-volume loops obtained in an animal using MRI under 4 conditions: control and reduced loading, both without and with enhanced contractile state. Oblique lines indicate the end-systolic pressure-volume relations (ESPVR), intercepting with the line P = 80 mmHg to give V_{80} (see text).

Ventricular volume measurement by the conductance catheter was performed as described previously [6], but using the double-field configuration to improve linearity and accuracy of the method [18,19]. Briefly, two electric fields with opposite polarity and different strengths are set up in the LV cavity using the outermost pair of electrodes in the apex and the aorta. The remaining electrodes are used to measure five intraventricular conductances which are converted to LV volume using previously developed algorithms, using a Leycom Sigma-5-D signal conditioner-processor (CardioDynamics, Leiden, Netherlands). To obtain volumes in an absolute sense, a 3 ml bolus of 10% saturated hypertonic saline was injected into the pulmonary artery, thus changing the conductivity of the intraventricular blood transiently. This transient is used to calculate the parallel conductance of the structures surrounding the LV cavity [6], as previously described [20]. The calibration procedures were repeated with each intervention to avoid possible problems with dependence of parallel conductance on the size of the ventricle [21]. Pressure-volume loops were displayed continuously on an X-Y oscilloscope. The analog signals of ECG, LV pressure and total conductance volume were digitized with 12-bit accuracy at a sample frequency of 200 Hz and stored on hard disk for later analysis using a special software program (Leycom Conduct PC) on an IBM-compatible PC.

Study design

P-V loops were obtained by registering LV pressure simultaneously with LV volume, either obtained with MRI or with the conductance catheter. To obtain loops at different loading conditions, vascular resistance and preload were lowered by intravenous sodium nitroprusside (3-6 μg/kg/min). The effect of the dilatation was a decrease in systolic LV pressure of roughly 30 mmHg.

After the baseline data had been obtained using the above change in loading conditions, the nitroprusside infusion was maintained while dobutamine was administered at a rate of 10 mg/kg/min. This dosage is sufficient to override the negative inotropic effect of the beta blockade by metoprolol [22]. Subsequently, nitroprusside infusion was discontinued and after its load-reducing effects had disappeared, P-V loops were recorded once more while maintaining the dobutamine infusion. Again, ESPVR and PRSW were constructed and computed from the loops during the enhanced inotropic state. Data acquisition was not started until after steady state had been reached as monitored by LV pressure and ECG. During such steady states, volume data were recorded with the conductance catheter over a 15 min period in order to allow comparison with the results of MR imaging, where data acquisition requires 10-15 min.

The P-V loop by conductance catheter was obtained by averaging the data over this 15 min period. This procedure is essentially the same as followed previously in our laboratory [23]. Upon completion of the experiments, all catheters and sheaths were removed and the animals were allowed to recover in order to be used for subsequent studies.

Data analysis

In all of the measurement series, end-systolic pressure (ESP) and -volume (ESV) as well as end-diastolic volume (EDV) and ejection fraction (EF) were determined, as was heart rate and cardiac output. After determining the upper left hand corner of the P-V loops, the ESPVR was constructed by connecting these two points (Figure 1). The slope, E_{es}, of the relationship was computed. Rather than extrapolating these lines to zero pressure to obtain V_d, a horizontal line was drawn at P = 80 mmHg to obtain V_{80}, because such a volume intercept in our opinion reflects the position of the ESPVR better than V_d in view of the nonlinearity of the relationship [23]. Either an increased slope or a decreased volume intercept or both reflect an increased inotropic state of the ventricle [2,3]. A leftward shift of the ESPVR was quantified by the change in V_{80}, and the increase in slope, E_{es}, was quantified by the ratio of its values before and after dobutamine. Statistical significance was tested using the sign test for change ; differences were considered significant at $p<0.01$.

Results

Most of the results reported here have been published previously [24,25]. A typical example of P-V loops obtained with MR imaging is given in Figure 1. Note that data points are shown only during ejection and part of the isovolumic relaxation phase because of limitations in the number of images that could be acquired. However, sufficient details are available to determine the end-systolic P-V points and, thus, the ESPVR. Clearly, dobutamine administration resulted in a leftward shift (notice the line revealing the volume intercept, V_{80}) as well as an increased slope of the relationship. The hemodynamic data obtained from the conductance catheter as well as MRI are given in Table 1.

Table 1: Hemodynamic effects of nitroprusside and dobutamine

	ESP mmHg	ESV ml	EDV ml	EF %	HR min^{-1}	CO l/min
cond.cath.						
control	103±4	21±2.1	47±2.2	57±2.7	88±4	2.4±.17
nitropruss.	70±3	13±2.2	37±2.8	65±3.6	88±5	2.0±.15
dobutamine	102±5	12±1.3	33±1.5	63±3.6	127±6	2.6±.12
dobu. + nitro.	77±4	8±1.0	24±1.8	70±2.2	133±6	2.2±.15
MRI						
control	96±3	25±2.5	60±2.7	59±2.5	85±4	3.0±.08
nitropruss.	68±2	17±1.9	48±2.7	69±2.9	97±6	3.1±.08
dobutamine	98±3	18±1.5	50±2.1	64±2.1	113±5	3.6±.17
dobu. + nitro.	73±3	12±1.0	35±2.2	71±2.2	125±5	3.1±.18

Shown are mean values ± SEM. During dobutamine, dP/dt_{max}, measured during conductance experiments (not shown), increased significantly ($p<0.01$), indicating increased contractility.

The table reveals the following:

1) Nitroprusside lowers systolic LV pressure by about 30 mmHg, statistically significant at $p<0.01$. It also lowers ESV and EDV, reflecting a decrease in preload, while cardiac output is hardly affected. Ejection fraction is slightly increased, which is due to the decrease in afterload. Heart rate is unchanged. After dobutamine, these changes by nitroprusside are maintained.

2) Dobutamine does not increase LV systolic pressure, but increased heart rate substantially in the dosage used. The drug decreased ESV as well as EDV while increasing EF and CO slightly.

3) The systolic pressure values in the MRI experiments are somewhat lower than in the conductance experiments, which is due to the time lapse between the measurement series and the gradual and unavoidable degradation of the preparation.

4) The volume and CO values obtained by conductance catheter are almost invariably smaller than those obtained by MRI. This phenomenon will be discussed below.

The ESPVR obtained in all experiments are shown in Figure 2. The dotted lines are drawn at $P = 80$ mmHg to give the values of V_{80} by intersection with the ESPVR in

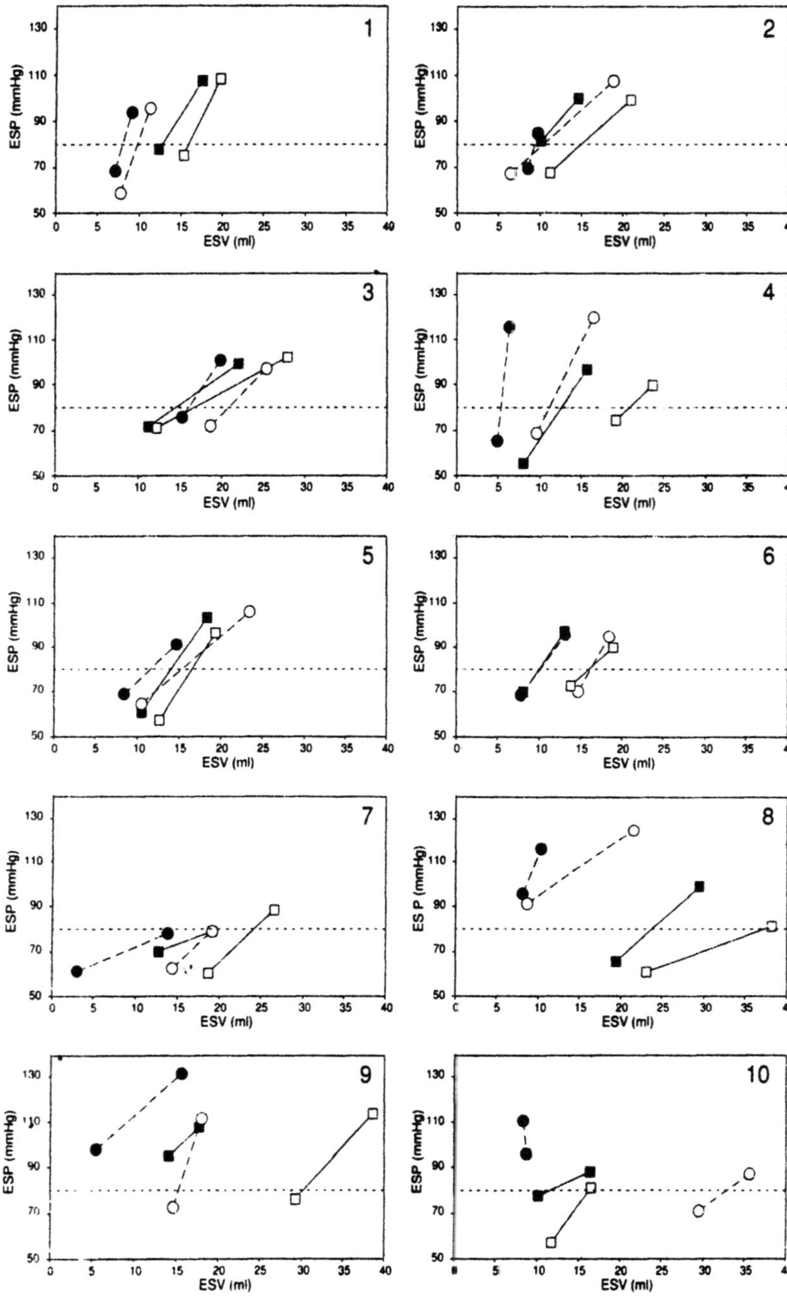

Fig. 2: ESPVRs in 10 anesthetized piglets, obtained using load reduction (nitroprusside), with MRI (solid lines, squares) and with conductance catheter (dashed lines, circles). Open squares and circles represent basal inotropic state, closed symbols represent increased inotropism by dobutamine. ESP resp. ESV: end-systolic pressure, resp. volume.

most cases. In a few instances such as animal 8 for the conductance measurements and animal 9 for MRI and conductance measurements after dobutamine, the relationships were extrapolated slightly to obtain V_{80}. The figure shows in general the same trends as noted above, but more specifically: in all animals, the ESPVR obtained with MRI during dobutamine showed a clear leftward shift compared to the control relation. The average leftward shift of the V_{80} values is 6.9 ml, highly significant at $p<0.002$. The slope of the relationship sometimes shows an increase, sometimes a decrease, but on the average, it did not change, as shown in Figure 3. For the conductance experiments, the ESPVR showed a similar leftward shift after dobutamine in all animals except nr.2 in which there was no change and nr. 10 where the dobutamine ESPVR probably indicates an artifact in the volume measurement. On the average, the decrease in V_{80} with dobutamine is 7.4 ml (Figure 3), which is rather close to the decrease obtained with MRI. In all animals except nrs. 9 and 10, the change in the slope or the absence thereof is similar for the conductance and the MRI measurements. On the average, there was no change in slope with the conductance experiments as shown in Figure 3. Statistically the changes in the slopes were not significant for either volume registration method.

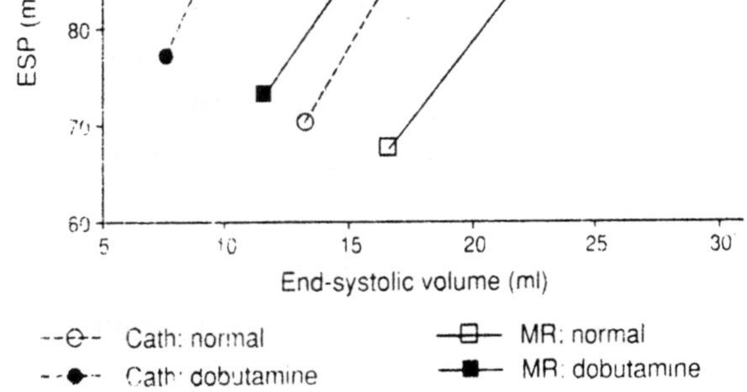

Fig. 3: Mean ESPVRs averaged for all animals, obtained by MRI (solid lines, squares) and by conductance catheter (dashed lines, circles), before (open symbols) and after dobutamine (solid symbols). Enhanced inotropism resulted in almost parallel shift of the ESPVR to smaller volume intercept at 80 mmHg.

Discussion

The study shows that pressure-volume loops may be obtained reliably both during normal and decreased loading conditions using magnetic resonance imaging, provided a special micromanometer tip catheter is used to minimize imaging artifacts. By connecting the end-systolic P-V points, the end-systolic pressure-volume relation may be constructed in a straightforward fashion. By increasing the contractile state of the heart by dobutamine infusion, these relations showed, on the average, a leftward shift without an increase in slope. Such behavior has been reported previously in animal studies using the conductance method or sonomicrometry [8,26,27]. In most of these studies, the increase in slope of the ESPVR was either small or absent. Furthermore, the leftward shift, as quantified by the value of V_{80}, was similar for the MRI and the conductance measurements. The fact that all volume values of the latter were smaller than those obtained by MRI reflects the well-known fact that the conductance catheter tends to underestimate true volume if the slope factor (α) is assumed to be 1 as was done in this study. In reality this factor is about 0.8 for dogs of the same size as the piglets [6]. For a quantity such as the ejection fraction its value is of no importance and indeed, table 1 reveals EF values very similar for the two methods.

The conductance catheter has, however, the great advantage over the MRI method in that it can register hemodynamic and drug-induced changes in performance instantaneously, i.e. on a beat-to-beat basis. MRI, on the other hand, provides accurate volume estimates of the left ventricle noninvasively, and may be used also for similar measurement of the right ventricle [28]. The present study shows that the LV volume data may be combined with LV pressure to give at least the systolic and early diastolic portion of the P-V loop. However, for pressure measurement one still must insert an intraventricular catheter. In principle, it may be possible to substitute arterial systolic pressure, measured by e.g. the arm cuff method, for end-systolic LV pressure [29]. For other relationships also shown to reflect inotropic state, such as the slopes of the dP/dt_{max} vs. end-diastolic volume [4] and preload recruitable stroke work [5], however, LV pressure is a prerequisite.

The main advantage of the above pressure-volume relations and derived indices is their minimal dependency on loading conditions [27]. A striking example of such dependency of the popular index ejection fraction is given in the present study: table 1 shows that nitroprusside-mediated lowering of loading conditions increased EF by the same amount as dobutamine-mediated enhanced inotropism. A similar shortcoming of EF in comparison to the end-systolic stress-volume ratio to assess contractile function (in mitral regurgitation) has been shown by others [30].

It may be concluded that assessment of LV pump function and contractility by the use of pressure-volume relations obtained by MRI as well as by conductance catheter is feasible. The method shows promise for application in humans for diagnosis of diminished cardiac performance, due to e.g. coronary artery disease. Provided that satisfactory means are established to combine noninvasively measured pressure with the MRI data, routine assessment of pressure-volume relations, not only during load changes, but also during e.g. dobutamine stress-testing [31] comes within reach.

References

1. Grossman W, Lorell BH, editors. Diastolic relaxation of the heart. Boston: Martinus Nijhoff, 1988.
2. Suga H, Sagawa K. Instantaneous pressure-volume relationships and their ratio in the excised, supported canine left ventricle. Circ Res 1974;35:117-26.
3. Baan J, van der Velde ET, Steendijk P. Ventricular pressure-volume relations in vivo. Eur Heart J 1992;13: Suppl E:2-6.
4. Little WC. The left ventricular dP dtmax-end-diastolic volume relation in closed-chest dogs. Circ Res 1985;56:808-15.
5. Glower DD, Spratt JA, Snow ND, et al. Linearity of the Frank-Starling relationship in the intact heart: the concept of preload recruitable stroke work. Circulation 1985;71:994-1009.
6. Baan J, van der Velde ET, de Bruin HG, et al. Continuous measurement of left ventricular volume in animals and humans by conductance catheter. Circulation 1984;70:812-23.
7. Van Bel F, Steendijk P, Teitel DF, de Winter PJ, van der Velde ET, Baan J. Cerebral blood flow velocity: the influence of myocardial contractility on the velocity waveform of brain supplying arteries. Ultrasound Med Biol 1992;18:441-9.
8. Teitel DF, Klautz RJM, Steendijk P, van der Velde ET, van Bel F, Baan J. The end-systolic pressure-volume relationship in the newborn lamb: effects of loading and inotropic interventions. Pediatr Res 1991;29:473-82.
9. Leatherman GF, Shook TL, Leatherman SM, Colucci WS. Use of a conductance catheter to detect increased left ventricular inotropic state by end-systolic pressure-volume analysis. Basic Res Cardiol 1989;84: Suppl 1:247-56.
10. Kass DA, Maughan WL. From 'Emax' to pressure-volume relations: a broader view. Circulation 1988;77:1203-12.
11. Baur LHB, Schipperheyn JJ, Baan J, et al. Influence of angiotensin converting enzyme inhibition on pump function and cardiac contractility in patients with chronic congestive heart failure. Br Heart J 1991;65:137-42.
12. Baan J. Evaluation of left ventricular dysfunction by pressure-volume loops. In Baur LHB, et al., editors. Opsporing en behandeling van een gestoorde linker-kamerfunctie na het myocardinfarct. Leiden: Boerhaave Commissie voor Postacademisch Onderwijs in de Geneeskunde, 1993:103-15.
13. Dell'Italia LJ, Carter B, Millar H, Pohost GM. Development of a micromanometer-tip catheter to record high-fidelity pressures during cine-gated NMR without significant image distortion. Magn Reson Med 1991;17: 119-25.

14. Pirolo JS, Branham BH, Cresswell LL, Perman WH, Vannier MW, Pasque MK. Pressure-gated acquisition of cardiac MR images. Radiology 1992;183:487-92.
15. Pattynama PMT, van der Velde ET, Steendijk P, Lamb HJ, Baan J, de Roos A. Cardiovascular MR imaging: pressure-gating using the arterial pressure signal from a conventional ferromagnetic micromanometer-tip catheter. Magn Res Imaging 1994;12:531-4.
16. Pattynama PMT, Lamb HJ, van der Velde EA, van der Wall EE, de Roos A. Left ventricular measurements with cine and spin-echo MR imaging: a study of reproducibility with variance component analysis. Radiology 1993; 187:261-8.
17. Press WH, Teukolsky SA, Vetterling WT, Flannery BP. Numerical recipes in C: the art of scientific computing: second edition. Cambridge: Cambridge University Press, 1992.
18. Steendijk P, van der Velde ET, Baan J. Single and dual excitation of the conductance-volume catheter analyzed in a spheroidal mathematical model of the canine left ventricle. Eur Heart J 1992;13 Suppl E:28-34.
19. Steendijk P, van Der Velde ET, Baan J. Left ventricular stroke volume by single and dual excitation of the conductance catheter in dogs. Am J Physiol 1993;264:H2189-207.
20. Baan J, van der Velde ET, Steendijk P, Koops J. Calibration and application of the conductance catheter for ventricular volume measurement. Automedica 1989;11:357-65.
21. Boltwood CM Iv, Appleyard RF, Glantz SA. Left ventricular volume measurement by conductance catheter in intact dogs. Parallel conductance volume depends on left ventricular size. Circulation 1989;80:1360-77.
22. Baan J, van der Velde ET. Sensitivity of left ventricular end-systolic pressure-volume relation to type of loading intervention in dogs. Circ Res 1988;62:1247-58.
23. Van der Velde ET, Burkhoff D, Steendijk P, Karsdon J, Sagawa K, Baan J. Nonlinearity and afterload sensitivity of end-systolic pressure-volume relation of canine left ventricle in vivo. Circulation 1991;83:315-27.
24. Pattynama PMT. Functional magnetic resonance imaging of the heart [Dissertation]. Leiden: Leiden University, 1994
25. Pattynama PMT, de Roos A, van der Velde ET, Lamb HJ, Steendijk P, Baan J. Magnetic resonance analysis of left ventricular pressure-volume relations: validation with the conductance method at rest and during dobutamine stress. Magn Reson Med. In press.
26. Van Bel F, Klautz RJM, Schipper IB, Teitel DF, Baan J. Autoregulatory ability of cerebral circulation before and after indomethacin in the newborn lamb [abstract]. Pediatr Res 1991;29:364A.
27. Little WC, Cheng CP, Peterson T, Vinten-Johansen J. Response of the left ventricular end-systolic pressure-volume relation in conscious dogs to a wide range of contractile states. Circulation 1988;78:736-45.
28. Longmore DB, Kl;ipstein RH, Underwood SR, et al. Dimensional accuracy of magnetic resonance in studies of the heart. Lancet 1985;1:1360-2.
29. Borow KM, Neumann A, Wynne J. Sensitivity of end-systolic pressure-dimension and pressure-volume relations to the inotropic state in humans. Circulation 1982;65:988-97.
30. Carabello BA, Nolan SP, McGuire LB. Assessment of preoperative left ventricular function in patients with mitral regurgitation: value of the end-systolic wall stress-end-systolic volume ratio. Circulation 1981;64:1212-7.
31. Van Rugge FP, van der Wall EE, Spanjersberg SJ, et al. Magnetic resonance imaging during dobutamine stress for detection and localization of coronary artery disease. Quantitative wall motion analysis using a modification of the centerline method. Circulation 1994;90:127-38.

Spectroscopy of the human heart: techniques, limitations and opportunities

P.R. Luyten[1]
Philips Medical Systems, Best, the Netherlands

Summary

Localized spectroscopy of the human heart offers a unique tool to study the biochemistry of the human myocardium in a non invasive and non destructive way. The technique has progressed steadily, using both advanced processing and data acquisition schemes to improve the reliability of the methodology. In spite of this progress, ^{31}P cardiac spectroscopy is still in the clinical research phase. If and when it will progress into routine clinical practice is unclear. More technique development (coil sensitivity, motion compensation, prior knowledge) and standardization will be required before this technique has matured in a diagnostic tool. In the mean time, as a research tool, localized spectroscopy of the human heart will remain a unique window to study cardiac metabolism.

Introduction

In vivo magnetic resonance spectroscopy (MRS) in humans was initiated by the measurement of in vivo phosphorous signals in muscle tissue. These first measurements have been directed towards the assessment of muscle metabolism using surface coils to localize the spectral information to a confined region of interest. All information acquired was confined within a small sensitive region close to the antenna that was used to receive the MRS signal. As subcutaneous fat does not produce a very clearly visible

[1] The author would like to acknowledge Jan den Hollander, Rolf Lamerichs, Biek Oosterwaal, Ron de Beer, Dik van Ormondt, Abert de Roos and Joost Doornbos for their contributions to the results described in this article.

E. E. van der Wall et al. (eds.), Advances in Imaging Techniques in Ischemic Heart Disease 71–81.

^{31}P MRS signal, all signal was derived from the musculature close to the coil that was used. The spectral information contained data on tissue composition in terms of several compounds that carry one or more ^{31}P nuclei. Phosphocreatine .(PCr), adenosine triphosphate (ATP) and inorganic phosphate (Pi) are the most important compounds that can be measured using this technique. Qualitative changes in the ratio of these peaks and the (absolute) determination of the intracellular pH gives information about the high energy phosphate metabolism and is indicative for the metabolic fate of normal and diseased tissue during stress tests. These pilot studies indicated already two decades ago that magnetic resonance is an unique technique to acquire metabolic information from living tissue in a non-invasive and non-destructive way. With the advent of localization techniques, in vivo whole body phosphorous spectroscopy could be used to study metabolism in other regions of the human body as well. Localized brain spectra have been used to study the metabolic changes in intracranial tumors, stroke, epilepsy, hepatic encephalopathy, white matter disorders and other pathologies that can be detected in the central nervous system. Liver and heart phosphorous spectroscopy have resulted in metabolic information under stress and ischemic conditions.

In spite of the matured localization techniques for spatially selective phosphorous spectroscopy, the clinical efficacy of these techniques is hampered by a number of physical limitations. First of all, phosphorous spectroscopy is an eternal struggle for better signal to noise ratio. Volumes of interest smaller than 10 cc will usually result in excessive measurement times, excluding these techniques for very focal pathologies. The main cause for the limited use (and progress) of localized ^{31}P spectroscopy in the human heart is the fact that signal to noise even with the most advanced MR techniques is still marginal, and that the localization of spectral information from a moving target poses an additional problem. A forthcoming problem are the intrinsic long longitudinal relaxation times of ^{31}P signal (T_1 in the order of seconds) which prohibit rapid acquisitions schemes to increase signal to noise. Also, the synchronization of data acquisition with the beating heart by ECG triggering prolongs the experiment even more. In this respect one should even consider to use gating or more advanced technique to correct for respiratory motion.

Due to the higher intrinsic sensitivity of the proton signal, the absence of MR visible lipid signal in the brain, no severe motion artifacts and somewhat more favorable relaxation times, most clinical spectroscopic applications using spatially resolved spectroscopy have focused on the brain. The clearly visible signals of N acetyl aspartate (NAA, a "neuronal marker"), Creatine (Cr) and Choline (Cho), Lactate (Lac), Alanine

(Ala), Inositol (In) and to a lesser extent glutamate (Glu) and glutamine (Gln) have resulted in a large number of studies of brain disorders. These studies produced much more pronounced observations of abnormal metabolism than analogous ^{31}P studies. Also, the higher sensitivity resulted in the application of spectroscopic imaging techniques that resolve the metabolic composition of the brain at a much higher spatial resolution (typically 0.5 - 2.0 cc)

The use of proton spectroscopy for cardiac applications in humans have been restricted to the detection of increased lipid signals associated with ischemic conditions of the myocardium [1] . As these studies may have a large potential in detecting compromised myocardial tissue, the problem of separating the myocardial lipids from the pericardial fat are phenomenal. All other human cardiac studies have used the ^{31}P signal. Applications have been reported for hypertrophic and dilated cardiomyopathies, left ventricular hypertrophy, valvular disease, transplanted hearts, myocardial infarctions and reversible ischemia (In a recent review article the different applications of cardiac spectroscopy have been described in more detail [2].)

Techniques: Spatial localization (MRS)

Several attempts have been made to derive information from the high energy metabolism in the human myocardium by using spatially resolved MR spectroscopy. The spatially resolution comprised techniques that:

1. obtain information from a single volume positioned around the anterior ventricular wall;
2. obtain information from a one-dimensional stack of slices that intersect the chest wall and consecutive slices through the myocardium. This stack may be spatially restricted in the two other dimensions;
3. obtain information of a fully three-dimensionally resolved data set.

The first reports on the clinical use of ^{31}P spectroscopy of the human heart clearly showed the result of underestimating the potential misinterpretations that can occur when using compromised localization techniques in a small, moving target. The problem with measuring "clean" myocardial spectra is aggravated by the fact that the myocardium is close to both the intercostal musculature and the ventricular blood. Both compartments have ^{31}P spectra which are almost similar to the spectrum of the myocardium. The intercostal muscle spectrum differs only from the myocardial spectra in the apparent PCr/ATP ratio and PCr/Pi ratio, whereas blood does have ATP signals, strong 2,3 diphosphoglycerate (2,3 DPG) signals and some serum phospholipid signal in the phosphomonoester region (Figure 1). Strong contamination of myocardial signal from blood or musculoskeletal signal may easily cause misinterpretation of the heart spectra. Initial reports of abnormal ^{31}P spectra in patients suffering from dilated cardiomyopathy could be explained by the substantial blood contamination in spectra taken from thin sections of myocardium in these patients. The signal in the mono- and diester regions of the spectrum originate from blood in the left ventricle. Still, after correcting for blood contamination and saturation effects, spectra in these patients show abnormalities in the PCr/ATP ratio [3].

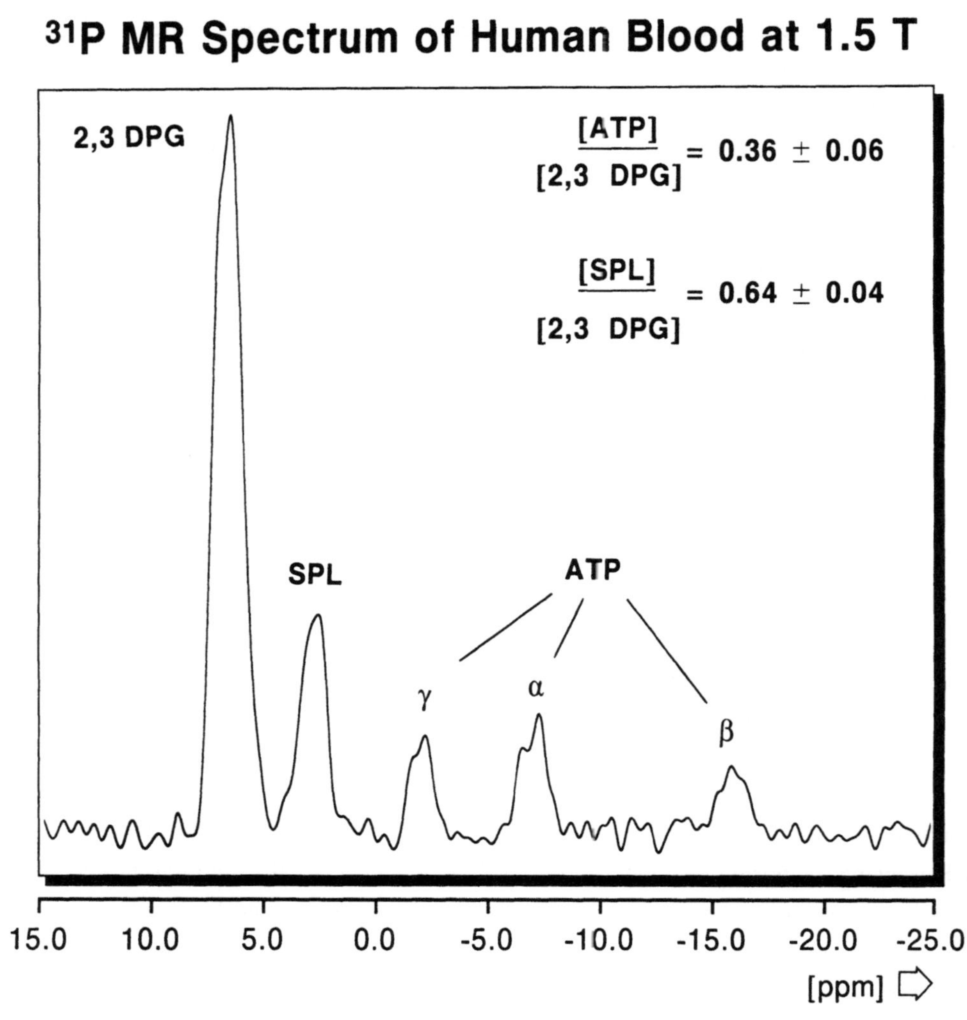

Fig. 1: Ex vivo ^{31}P spectrum of human blood at 1.5 T.

Presently, localization is obtained either by a fully three-dimensional spatial localization by phase encoding techniques only, or a one-dimensional phase encoding technique combined with two-dimensional column selection. The first technique has the advantage that the volumes obtained are isotropic. A problem may be caused by substantial motion artifacts, which result in poorly defined spectra in which the contamination of neighboring voxel is substantial. The latter technique may result in irregularly shaped volumes, but is susceptible to motion artifacts in the phase encoding dimension in one direction only. The volume selection is obtained by a two-dimensional column (slice) selection. Usually, 32 phase encoding steps are used with a field of view of 320 mm, resulting in 10 mm slices through the myocardium. As signal to noise requires multiple averages for the individual phase encoding steps, for the zeroth order profile typically 32 acquisitions may be acquired; for higher order profiles, that number is reduced following a cos or $\cos^2$ window to reduce finite sampling artifacts [4]. Figure 2 shows an example of a stack of spectra measured in a patient with dilated cardiomyopathy. An experiment like this will take approximately 25 minutes. (Typical TR is 3 seconds). From these results it is clearly shown how the spectra from the chest wall differ from spectra from the myocardium.

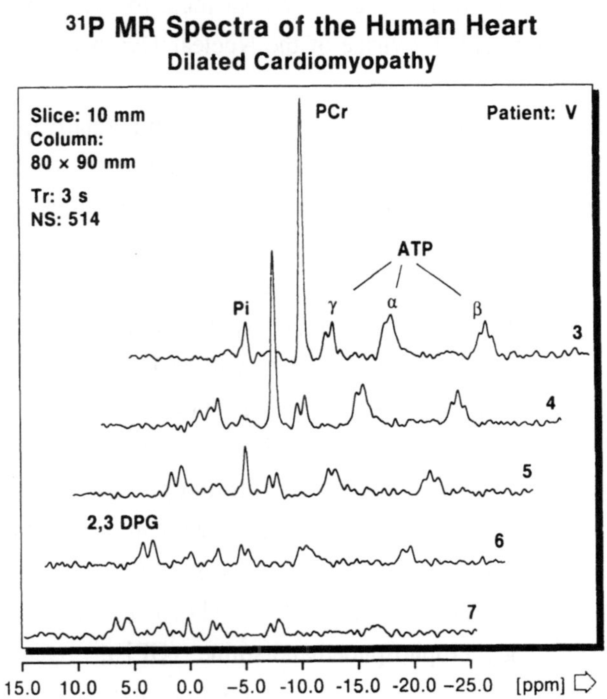

Fig. 2: Stack of ^{31}P spectra of 1 cm slices through the myocardium of a patient with hypertrophic cardiomyopathy.

Technique: Improving signal to noise by hetero nuclear decoupling

Higher field strengths may be advantageous to perform spectroscopy experiments due to the improved signal to noise. However, the line width of in vivo NMR signals is largely determined by tissue susceptibility which results in broader lines at higher field strengths. This effect limits the advantages of increasing the field strengths. Another reason for poor ^{31}P signal detection is the low intensity for some ^{31}P resonances due to complex J coupling patterns with protons. Further complications may result from the overlap of resonance frequencies between different components. Particularly the proton coupled 2,3 DPG signal may obscure the Pi signal.

One technique which may alleviate the signal to noise limitations at lower field strengths (1.5 - 2.0 T) to some extent is the use of proton decoupling in combination with whole body ^{31}P spectroscopy [5]. Proton decoupling may simplify the structure of the spectrum by suppressing the hetero nuclear J modulation patterns with the spin-spin coupled protons. E.g., proton decoupling will simplify the 2,3 DPG signal into a doublet, improving the conspicuity of the Pi signal. Moreover, excitation or saturation of the surrounding protons in the tissue may contribute to the signal strength of the individual phosphorous signals by virtue of the Nuclear Overhauser Effect (NOE).

As the J coupling between protons and phosphorous nuclei is relatively small, excellent shimming over the region of interest is an absolute necessity for good in vivo spectral resolution. Depending on the relevant tissue susceptibility and volume of interest size, a homogeneity of 0.05 - 0.3 ppm (full width at half maximum) can be achieved. Methods to accomplish this homogeneity either employ the spatially resolved water signal in an iterative shim process or generate B_0 maps obtained from phase sensitive imaging methods. After shimming the line width will be 1.5 - 7 Hz at 1.5 T for in vivo ^{31}P NMR resonances. These line widths are sufficient to resolve the homo nuclear ^{31}P J couplings of $\pm$ 17 Hz between the three nuclear ^{31}P spins of ATP. Since the 3 bond isotropic hetero nuclear coupling between protons and phosphorous is in the order of 6 - 10 Hz, this coupling may become the dominant factor in the residual resonance line width of ^{31}P nuclei coupled to one or more protons, such as in 2,3-diphosphoglycerate (2,3-DPG), nicotinamide adenine dinucleotide (NAD+), phosphoethanolamine (PE), phosphocholine (PC), glycerophosphoethanolamine (GPE), glycerophosphocholine (GPC) and alpha ATP. Therefore, proton decoupling at a field strength of 1.5 T combined with an excellent local homogeneity can improve spectral resolution substantially, resulting in more resolved resonances and more reliable quantitative information. At higher field strengths proton decoupling of ^{31}P MR signals will be less effective due to the increased line widths which may become larger than the actual J couplings.

Irradiation of protons during in vivo ^{31}P spectroscopy results in signal increase due to collapse of multiplet structures into singlets. Furthermore, this irradiation may introduce NOE which also results in significant signal increase. This signal enhancement not only affects ^{31}P nuclei which are coupled to protons within the same molecule. Also, non-coupled resonances, e.g. the phosphocreatine (PCr) signal, may show a substantial increase in signal intensity during saturation of the surrounding water protons. Due to the hetero nuclear dipolar relaxation mechanism and the long dipolar cross relaxation times between the ^{31}P and ^{1}H water nuclei, the NOE may be quite effective. Similar to decoupling, the NOE may result in relatively larger signal enhancements at lower field strengths. This is related to the inherent relaxation mechanisms for the ^{31}P nuclear spins. The two most important relaxation mechanisms for in vivo ^{31}P signals originate either from dipolar interactions or from the shielding anisotropy. Because this latter relaxation mechanism is proportional to B_0^2, it becomes the predominant relaxation mechanism at higher field strengths, resulting in a decreased NOE.

A variety of effective pulse sequences have been developed for decoupling purposes, especially for high resolution MR applications. A well defined decoupling sequence requires a homogeneous decoupling field B_1 which exceeds the strength of the J couplings involved and covers the entire spectral range of the proton spectrum that has to be decoupled. Broad band decoupling techniques generally rely on repeated inversion of the proton spins. Therefore, they require inversion pulses with a repetition time short compared to 1/J. For proton decoupling of in vivo ^{31}P NMR signals, these conditions are easily fulfilled with the current 1.5 T whole body technology. First of all, the J coupling involved are very small, only in the order of 6 - 10 Hz. This allows for relatively long pulses, and concomitantly for low radiofrequency (rf) power levels to decouple sufficiently. Furthermore, the relevant in vivo proton resonances coupled to phosphorous nuclei resonate in a small chemical shift range of $\pm$ 100 Hz around the H_2O resonance. This again allows for low rf power without affecting the broadband decoupling performance. Sufficient decoupling power can be generated utilizing a WALTZ-4 sequence using a basic 90 degree pulse length of 900 μs, corresponding to an expected decoupling band width of $\pm$ 280 Hz around the water resonance. These values allow for the use of large resonators such as standard whole body ^{1}H transmission coils employed on clinical MR scanners. For NOE the conditions are even more favorable. As most NOE contributions are expected to originate from the tissue water only, a low power single frequency irradiation of the water protons can be sufficient to generate large NOE enhancements.

As the availability of second rf channels on clinical 1.5 T scanners is still limited, the number of in vivo applications is quite restricted. However, for all applications of ^{31}P MRS, especially for studies on focal pathologies, proton decoupling showed an important improvement in the sensitivity of the technique. A nuclear Overhauser enhancement factor for PCr of 0.74 can easily be obtained. (Signal increase of 1.74) For purely ^{31}P-^{1}H dipolar relaxation and under extreme narrowing conditions the maximum enhancement factor is given by $\eta = \gamma(^{1}H)/2\,\gamma(^{31}P) = 1.24$. This implies, that combined broad band decoupling during acquisition and single frequency low power irradiation at the water resonance frequency during all relaxation delays results in a substantial signal increase. This effect however may have an important impact on the quantification of ^{31}P MR signals which are obtained using double resonance techniques. So all reports on quantitative ^{31}P spectroscopy should indicate the typical enhancement factors obtained by proton decoupling to assess the outcome of the study.

Techniques: quantification

One crucial step towards clinically useful cardiac spectroscopy is the ability to quantitate the spectra. A first prerequisite to quantitate in vivo ^{31}P spectra is the reliability of the localization technique. Even with excellent signal to noise and very sophisticated numerical data fitting routines, absolute quantification of metabolite levels in the myocardium will be extremely difficult. The problems to overcome are:

- B1 inhomogeneity of the surface coil(s) will require an accurate calibration procedure to compensate for the decrease in sensitivity further away from the coil. Especially when the size of the measured volume is in the same order of magnitude as the radius of the coil, sensitivity changes over the measured slice or volume itself will affect the measured signal intensity.

- The experimental conditions (pulse settings, partial saturation, partial decoupling and/or Overhauser enhancements) may strongly influence the obtained signal strength.

- Accurate quantification, either in frequency or time domain, may become a difficult problem for the relatively low signal to noise spectra measured in ^{31}P spectroscopy.

We have been using time domain fitting routine [6,7] using prior knowledge of the ^{31}P spectrum in terms of fixed values for the J-coupling patterns for the ATP signals, a fixed position for GPC and blood phospholipid signals, fixed amplitude and decay ratios for the three ATP signals and fixed line widths for the PDE, Pi and 2,3 DPG signals. This method was used to measure ratios of PCr, ATP and Pi metabolites and the absolute pH value in patients with dilated and hypertrophic cardiomyopathies.

Example of clinical use of ^{31}P cardiac spectroscopy

Figure 2 shows a stack of spectra taken from a patient with dilated cardiomyopathy. Slices 3 and 4 clearly represent ^{31}P spectra from the chest muscle, whereas slice 6 and 7 represent spectra from the anterior wall of the left ventricle. Spectrum 5 will be composed of a mixture of chest muscle and myocardium. To illustrate the difficulty in discriminating signal from the myocardium and the ventricular blood pool, a (deoxygenated) blood spectrum is shown in Figure 3. The broad lines are due to the deoxygenation, but still this experiment at 1.5 T using the same localization techniques as the clinical measurements gives an indication of the ratio between 2,3 DPG, the serum phospholipids and ATP. As the myocardium does not show 2,3 DPG, this signal can be used to estimate the blood contamination in the dilated cardiomyopathy spectrum as shown in Figure 3. Taking this correction and partial saturation effects into account, the PCr/ATP ratio for this particular case was found to be 0.62 ± 0.12 [3] The normal value for this ratio should be around 1.8 [2].

The data set in Figure 4 was obtained by time domain analysis of a set of cardiac ^{31}P spectra in a volunteer. The simulated data show another interesting phenomenon. In this stack of spectra the transition from the chest wall into the myocardium is clearly visible (slice 27) due to the shift in resonance frequency of the spectrum, resulting in a split PCr peak. This effect reflects different composition of both muscle types. Again this shows that ^{31}P spectroscopy in the human heart may resolve subtle effects in the biochemistry of the myocardium.

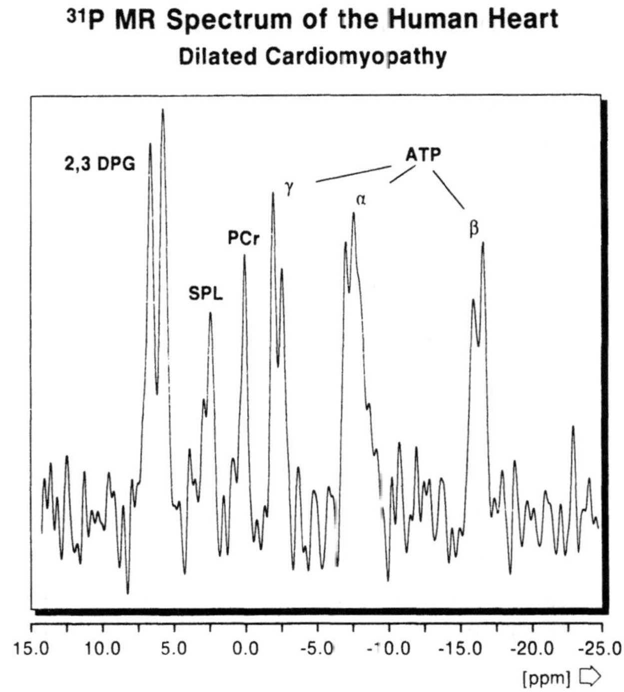

Fig. 3: The ^{31}P spectrum of a mixture of ventricular blood and human myocardium.

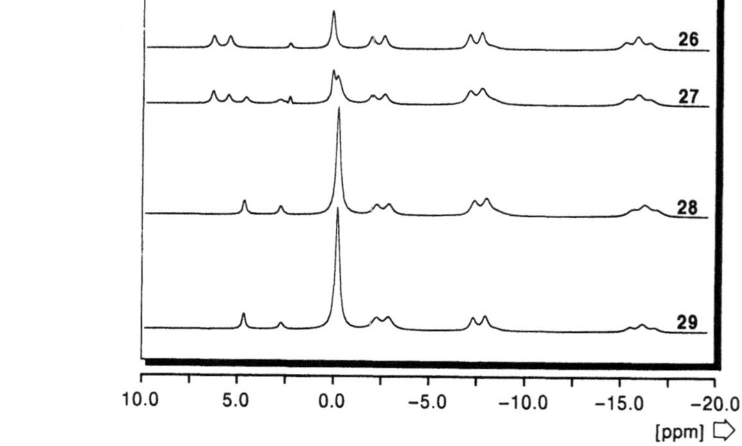

Fig. 4: Stack of processed ^{31}P spectra through the myocardium of a volunteer.

References

1. den Hollander JA, Evanochko WT, Pohost GM, Observation of cardiac lipids in humans by localized 1H magnetic resonance spectroscopic imaging. Magn Reson Med 1994;32:175-80.
2. Bottomley PA. MR spectroscopy of the human heart: the status and the challenges. Radiology 1994;191 :593-612.
3. de Roos A, Doornbos J, Luyten PR, Oosterwaal LJMP, van der Wall EE, den Hollander JA. Cardiac metabolism in patients with dilated and hypertrophic cardiomyopathy: assessment with proton-decoupled P-31 MR spectroscopy. J. Magn Reson Imaging 1992;2:711-9.
4. den Hollander JA, de Roos A, Doornbos J, Oosterwaal LJMP, Luyten PR. Practical aspects of in vivo 31P nuclear magnetic resonance spectroscopy of the human myocardium. In: Pohost GM, editor. Cardiovascular applications of magnetic resonance. Mount Kisco, NY: Futura Publishing Co., 1993; 403-16.
5. Luyten PR, Bruntink G, Sloff FM et al. Broadband proton decoupling in human ^{31}P NMR spectroscopy. NMR Biomed 1989;1:177-83.
6. van Ormondt D, de Beer R, Mariën AJH, den Hollander JA, Luyten PR, Vermeulen JWAH. 2D approach to quantification of inversion-recovery data. J Magn Reson 1990;88:652-9.
7. van der Veen JWC, de Beer R, Luyten P, van Ormondt D. Accurate quantification of in vivo ^{31}P NMR signals using the variable projection method and prior knowledge. Magn Reson Med 1988;6:92-8.

Current status of stress echocardiography for the diagnosis of myocardial ischemia and viability

Th.H. Marwick
Department of Cardiology, Cleveland Clinic International Center, U.S.A.

Summary

Stress echocardiography is now accepted as a routine technique for the investigation of coronary disease. The interpretation of stress echocardiograms for clinical purposes is currently performed using qualitative interpretation. Training on the part of the observer is very important from this standpoint. The accuracy of exercise echocardiography for the diagnosis of coronary artery disease is in the range of 85%, and for non exercise stress, it appears to be comparable, although patients who can exercise shoud do so, because exercise is a more vigorous form of stress than the pharmacological alternatives. Exercise echocardiography is more accurate than the exercise electrocardiogram, particularly in women and in patients with left ventricular hypertrophy. It appears to have a comparable accuracy to myocardial perfusion scintigraphy, being somewhat less sensitive than the latter although more specific. In addition to its diagnostic use stress echocardiography has been found to be useful for prognostic assessment of patients undergoing vascular surgery, patients following myocardial infarction, and those with chronic stable coronary disease. Finally, this technique has found attractive and interesting new uses in the evaluation of patients with possible viable myocardium, and patients with valvular heart disease.

Feasibility

Stress echocardiography has progressed from being a predominantly research technique carried out in a few centers, to being a routine technique for the investigation of coronary artery disease [1-5]. The underlying principle is that ischemic tissue

E. E. van der Wall et al. (eds.), Advances in Imaging Techniques in Ischemic Heart Disease 83–99.

demonstrates abnormalities in regional left ventricular function which are provoked by stress and correlate closely with the onset of ischemia.

As the technique is currently performed in routine clinical practice, it's interpretation is qualitative and therefore subjective. Table 1 summarizes the algorithm which is currently applied for the purposes of this interpretation. Most centers use a segmental left ventricular model in order to standardize this subjective methodology [6], most commonly the 16 segment model recommended by the American Society of Echocardiography, and score the function of each segment before, during and after stress (Figure 1). The stress echocardiography report should therefore include comments on global left ventricular function before and after stress (which may be quantitated if required), regional left ventricular function before and after stress (usually as a wall motion score), the site, extent, onset, duration, and severity of wall motion abnormalities before and after stress, and other cardiac diagnoses including the presence and severity of valvular and pericardial disease.

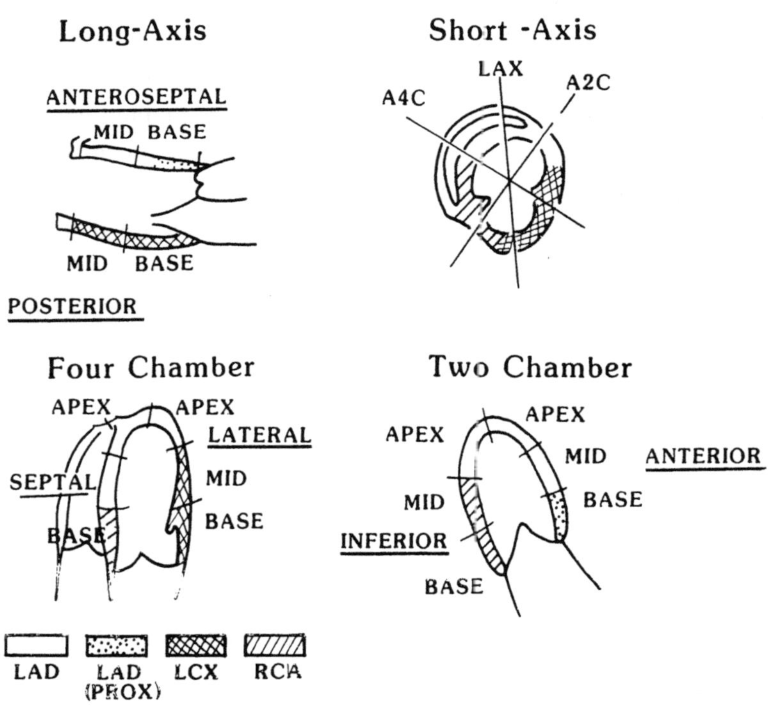

Fig. 1: Segmentation of the left ventricle for regional wall motion analysis.

Table 1: Qualitative interpretation of dubotamine echocardiography.

Diagnosis	Resting function	Low-dose	Peak/post-stress function
Normal	Normal	Normal	Hyperkinetic
Ischemic	Normal	Normal (unless severe CAD)	Reduction vs. rest Reduction vs. other segments Delayed contraction
Viable, patent IRA	Hypo/akinetic	Improvement	Sustained improvement
Viable, stenosed IRA	Hypo/akinetic	Improvement	Reduction c/w low-dose
Infarction	A/dyskinetic	No change	No change

The disadvantage of this qualitative approach is that a significant learning curve is required for both the sonographer and particularly the interpreting physician. The requisite duration is unclear, but it should involve about 100 studies over several months [7]. Although quantitative methods, involving the centerline technique, have been used in studies [8], they are too cumbersome and time-consuming for clinical practice using current technology. In addition, endocardial resolution, translational movement correction and automated methods of tracking the endocardial border all need to be improved before quantitative regional wall motion analysis becomes feasible clinically.

Accuracy of stress echocardiography

Exercise echocardiography

Provided that the stress echocardiograms are interpreted by experienced observers, the expected sensitivity and specificity which can be attained with the technique are in the 80-85% range (Table 2). It should be kept in mind that the values of sensitivity and specificity are highly dependent upon the population selected, and that the inclusion of patients with previous infarction, disproportionate numbers of patients with multi-vessel disease, and very aggressive reading of minor wall motion abnormalities all result in high sensitivities at the cost of lower specificities. While technically difficult or inadequate studies (obtained > 2 minutes after exercise) should be reviewed with caution, there are a few other predictors of inaccurate results. In our experience, the major predictors of false negatives were patients who exercised submaximally (to < 85% of age-predicted maximum), and patients with moderate stenoses (50-70% diameter) as well as those with single vessel coronary disease [9]. Anti-anginal therapy, if it prevents the heart from being stressed maximally, may cause false negative results [10].

Table 2: Sensitivity and specificity of digital exercise echocardiography for the diagnosis of CAD.

Author	Multivessel (% all CAD)	MI (% all CAD)	Sensitivity - overall	Sensitivity - SVD pts	Sensitivity MI excluded	Specificity
Armstrong, Ann Intern Med 1986	45 (56%)	36 (45%)	88% (n=80)	-	80% (n=44)	87% (n=15)
Armstrong, J Am Coll Cardiol 1987	59 (58%)	50 (50%)	88% (n=101)	81% (n=42)	78% (n=51)	86% (n=22)
Ryan, J Am Coll Cardiol 1988	15 (38%)	0	78% (n=40)	76% (n=25)	78% (n=40)	100% (n=24)
Sawada, J Am Coll Cardiol 1989	11 (39%)	0	86% (n=28)	88% (n=17)	86% (n=28)	86% (n=29)
Sheikh, J Am Coll Cardiol 1990	0	0	81% (n=21)	81% (n=21)	81% (n=21)	92% (n=13)
Crouse, Am J Cardiol 1991	106 (61%)	-	97% (n=175)	92% (n=66)	-	64% (n=53)
Pozzoli, Am J Cardiol 1991	16 (33%)	0	71% (n=49)	60% (n=33)	71% (n=49)	88% (n=26)
Marwick, J Am Coll Cardiol 1992	54 (47%)	55 (48%)	84% (n=114)	77% (n=60)	80% (n=59)	86% (n=36)
Salustri, Am Heart J 1992	0	0	86% (n=30)	86% (n=30)	86% (n=30)	64% (n=14)
Quinones, Circulation 1992	45 (52%)	-	74% (n=85)	58% (n=41)	-	81% (n=26)
Ryan, J Am Soc Echo 1993	126 (60%)	132 (63%)	91% (n=211)	86% (n=85)	95% (n=126)	78% (n=98)
Hecht, J Am Coll Cardiol 1993	82 (60%)	38 (28%)	93% (n=137)	84% (n=55)	100% (n=82)	86% (n=43)

Non-exercise echocardiography

The only factor which is predictive of an inaccurate result before the test is performed is submaximal exercise. The proportion of patients who are either unable to exercise or exercise submaximally varies from 35-40% in the stress laboratories of tertiary care institutions [11]. In this situation, a nonexercise stressor is appropriate. The choice for clinical practice falls between dobutamine, the coronary vasodilators dipyridamole and adenosine, and transesophageal atrial pacing. Each of these techniques is attended by disadvantages, but vasodilator stress is the least favored as this increases cardiac workload to a relatively small degree, and produces ischemia mainly through reduced coronary supply secondary to steal [12]. Transesophageal pacing can be relied upon to provide a sustained tachycardia, but often does not provoke hypertension, and may also not be well tolerated by the patient The accuracy of pharmacologic echocardiography for the diagnosis of coronary disease is summarized in Table 3. Generally, more recent studies of dobutamine echocardiography have shown sensitivities in the range of 80%, slightly lower than that obtained with exercise stress, with comparable specificities.

Table 3: Sensitivity and specificity of echocardiography with pharmacologic stress (studies of >50 patients).

Author	n	Stress technique	"Significant" stenosis dia	Multivessel (% all CAD)	M infarctn (% all CAD)	Sensitivity - overall	Sensitivity - SVD	Specificity
Cohen	50	Dipy 400mg po	>70%	28 (78%)	16 (44%)	81% (n=36)	88% (n=8)	93% (n=14)
Picano	93	Dipy 0.84mg/kg *	>70%	48 (67%)	17 (24%)	74% (n=72)	50% (n=12)	100% (n=21)
Marwick	97	Ad 0.18mcg/kg/min*	>50%	28 (47%)	0 (0%)	58% (n=59)	52% (n=31)	87% (n=38)
Mazeika	55	Dipy 1.00mg/kg *	>70%	30 (75%)	18 (45%)	40% (n=40)	0% (n=10)	93% (n=15)
Picano	66	Dipy 0.56mg/kg	>70%	20 (40%)	9 (18%)	56% (n=50)	37% (n=30)	100% (n=16)
Masini	83	Dipy 0.84mg/kg *	>70%	24 (62%)	15 (38%)	79% (n=39)	-	93% (n=44)
Picano	445	Dipy 0.84mg/kg *	>50%	119 (46%)	0 (0%)	96% (n=256)	56% (n=137)	96% (n=135)
Massa	52	Dipy 0.84mg/kg *	>70%	12 (23%)	9 (17%)	90% (n=52)	-	-
Pingitore	130	Dipy 0.84mg/kg+atr	>50%	-	-	87% (n=94)	-	94% (n=34)
Beleslin	136	Dipy 0.84mg/kg *	>50%	11 (9%)	41(34%)	74% (n=119)	72% (n=108)	94% (n=27)
Sawada	103	Dobu 30 mcg/kg/min	>50%	14 (40%)	35 (43%)	95% (n=81)	89% (n=38)	77% (n=22)
Cohen	70	Dobu 40 mcg/kg/min	>70%	35 (69%)	19 (37%)	86% (n=51)	69% (n=16)	95% (n=19)
Salustri	52	Dobu 40 mcg/kg/min	>50%	17 (46%)	14 (38%)	54% (n=37)	40% (n=20)	80% (n=15)
Marcowitz	141	Dobu 30 mcg/kg/min	>50%	47 (43%)	-	96% (n=109)	95% (n=62)	66% (n=32)
Mazeika	50	Dobu 20 mcg/kg/min	>70%	24 (67%)	13 (36%)	78% (n=36)	50% (n=12)	93% (n=14)
Marwick	217	Dobu 40 mcg/kg/min	>50%	74 (52%)	0 (0%)	72% (n=142)	66% (n=68)	83% (n=75)
Hoffman	66	Dobu 40 mcg/kg/min	>70%	21 (42%)	0 (0%)	79% (n=50)	78% (n=29)	87% (n=16)
McNeill	80	Dobu 40 mcg/kg/min+atro	>50%	15 (32%)	28 (60%)	70% (n=47)	-	88% (n=33)
Prince	81	Dobu 40 mcg/kg/min+TEE	>70%	16 (76%)	7 (33%)	90% (n=21)	100% (n=5)	94% (n=52)
Takeuchi	120	Dobu 30 mcg/kg/min	>50%	37 (50%)	62 (84%)	85% (n=74)	73% (n=37)	93% (n=46)
Beleslin	136	Dobu 40 mcg/kg/min	>50%	11 (9%)	41(34%)	82% (n=119)	82% (n=108)	77% (n=27)

* Low dose positivity permits conclusion of study before stated "peak" dose

Ad = adenosine, atr = atropine, dia = diameter of coronary artery, Dipy = dipyridamole, ex = exercise, M infarctn = myocardial infarction, SVD = single vessel disease, TEE = transesophageal echocardiography

Exercise vs non-exercise techniques

The performance of stress echocardiography during dobutamine stress is substantially easier than that during or following exercise stress, because the patient is stationary and not hyperventilating. As the technique is technically easier, some thought has been given to replacing exercise with dobutamine stress even in those patients who are able to exercise. While under optimal conditions, similar levels of sensitivity may be obtained using either technique [13-16], dobutamine is a less potent stress on the heart than exercise. As a consequence, when compared on a head-to-head basis, some patients with coronary disease may be detected with exercise but not with dobutamine stress. This is particularly a problem if the dobutamine is limited by side effects or the patient is beta blocked. Indeed, even if both exercise and dobutamine tests are positive, the extent of ischemia induced by exercise is significantly greater than that produced by dobutamine [17]. The consequence of this is that the interpreting physician may be more confident about the diagnosis of ischemia (as more extensive myocardial segments are demonstrated to be more abnormal) and this to an extent may balance the lower image quality of exercise compared with dobutamine stress.

Comparison with the stress ECG

The stress electrocardiogram is the most widely accepted and applied technique for non-invasive diagnosis of coronary disease. The comparison of the exercise ECG and exercise echo should be considered in 3 subgroups; patients in whom the exercise ECG is uninterpretable, patients who are unable to exercise, and those in whom maximal exercise is obtainable and the exercise ECG is interpretable. In those patients in whom the ECG is uninterpretable, the use of a stress imaging test (traditionally perfusion imaging) is widely accepted, and stress echocardiography is an accurate alternative [18]. In patients who have an interpretable electrocardiogram but are unable to exercise, the accuracy of dipyridamole or dobutamine stress electrocardiography is poor, with studies documenting a sensitivity of less than 50% for the identification of both single and multivessel coronary disease [19].

In the remaining patients, in whom maximal exercise is possible and the ST segment is interpretable, comparisons of the exercise echo and exercise ECG have repeatedly shown a benefit in favor of exercise echocardiography. Clearly, however, the widespread use of exercise echocardiography in place of the exercise ECG is not feasible from a logistic and financial standpoint. Consequently, it seems prudent to consider the routine practice of exercise echocardiography as a primary test in those particular patients who produce diagnostic problems for the exercise ECG alone. The first such group is women, in whom the specificity of the stress ECG is suboptimal [20]. Several studies have now shown a benefit in favor of exercise echocardiography with respect to specificity [21-23], and analysis of the cost of using exercise echocardiography as a primary test in this group has confirmed the approach to be cost effective, because of the avoidance of costly coronary angiography in patients who have false/positive stress ECG [23]. A second group of patients in whom the stress ECG is particularly unreliable are those with left ventricular hypertrophy. In this situation, the exercise echocardiogram is significantly more accurate, both when the hypertrophy is diagnosed electrocardiographically, and when it is suspected clinically.

In summary, stress echocardiography should be considered as a primary test in preference to the exercise ECG in patients who have uninterpretable ST segments, who are unable to exercise, and in women and patients with known or suspected left ventricular hypertrophy. It might be considered in patients who require both an exercise test and an echocardiogram, as an efficient and inexpensive way of getting both sets of data together. In other situations, where the patient is able to exercise maximally and the ECG is diagnostic, it should be realized that the stress echocardiography is significantly more accurate than the stress ECG, and might be used as a secondary test if the results of the routine stress test are inconsistent with the clinical status or nondiagnostic. This is not to say that the stress ECG should in any way be replaced by the stress echocardiogram. Patients are frequently sent for stress testing to examine parts of the stress response unrelated to the electrocardiogram, including their exercise capacity and the development of arrhythmias in response to exercise.

Comparison with myocardial perfusion scintigraphy

The use of stress-imaging combinations as a primary test in various situations has become accepted in recent years, and perfusion scintigraphy has traditionally fulfilled this role. The place of stress echocardiography in relation to perfusion scintigraphy is still being defined. Certainly, from a theoretical standpoint, it would be expected that as the development of flow heterogeneity necessarily preceeds the development of regional myocardial dysfunction, the sensitivity of the scintigram should exceed that of the stress echocardiogram. However, it should be remembered that the "ischemic cascade" was developed from data gathered from animal experiments involving a "supply side" rather than "demand side" pattern of ischemia. Moreover, these differences may be modulated by the technical limitations of myocardial perfusion imaging.

A review of the recent literature for myocardial perfusion scintigraphy demonstrates that using thallium SPECT, a sensitivity of >90% can be expected for the detection of significant coronary disease. However, the specificity of perfusion imaging in recent studies has been more of the order of 70%, due to both referral bias and artifacts during thallium imaging [24]. Moreover, there is substantial heterogeneity in the results obtained with myocardial perfusion imaging, just as there is with stress echocardiography, dependent on the nature of the patient population. Therefore, the techniques are most satisfactorily compared when they are performed in the same individuals. Unfortunately, if they are compared in the absence of a gold standard test, such as coronary angiography, it is impossible to discern which test result is correct, particularly when questions relate to the specificity of perfusion imaging.

The optimal study design for comparison of stress echocardiography and perfusion scintigraphy involves the performance of both tests in the same patients, with coronary angiography used as the arbitor of which test is correct. Several such studies are summarized in Table 4; these results demonstrate that the accuracy of both exercise and non-exercise echocardiography and perfusion scintigraphy are comparable, apart from when vasodilator stress echocardiography is used, because the latter approach is relatively insensitive [25].

Table 4: Comparison of sensitivity and specificity of echocardiography and myocardial perfusion imaging after various stressors for the detection of CAD.

Author	Significant stenosis	Stress methodology	Nuclear methodology	Sensitivity - echo	Sensitivity - nuclear	Sens-SVD - echo	Sens-SVD - nuclear	Specificity - echo	Specificity - nuclear
Maurer, Am J Cardiol 1981	>50%	Treadmill	Planar Tl	83% (n=23)	74% (n=23)	50% (n=6)	-	92% (n=13)	92% (n=13)
Parodi, Circulation 1989	>50%	Dipy 0.84mg/kg	SPECT-MIBI	73% (n=60)	77% (n=60)	-	-	84% (n=19)	84% (n=19)
Galanti, Am Heart J 1991	>70%	Upright bike	Planar Tl	93% (n=27)	100% (n=27	93% (n=14)	100% (n=14	96% (n=26)	92% (n=26)
Perin, Clin Nucl Med 1991	>50%	Dipy 0.56mg/kg	SPECT-Tl	58% (n=19)	95% (n=19)	-	-	100% (n=6)	50% (n=6)
Simonetti, Circulation 1991	>75%	Dipy 0.84mg/kg	Planar Tl	86% (n=22)	91% (n=22)	-	-	92% (n=13)	100% (n=13)
Pozzoli, Am J Cardiol 1991	>50%	Upright bike	SPECT-MIBI	71% (n=49)	84% (n=49)	60% (n=33)	82% (n=33)	96% (n=26)	88% (n=26)
Salustri, Am Heart J 1992	>50%	Upright bike	SPECT-MIBI/Tl	86% (n=30)	83% (n=30)	86% (n=30)	83% (n=30)	85% (n=14)	64% (n=14)
Quinones, Circulation 1992	>50%	Treadmill	SPECT-Tl	74% (n=86)	76% (n=86)	58% (n=41)	61% (n=41)	88% (n=26)	81% (n=26)
Marwick, J Am Coll Cardiol 19	>50%	Db 40mcg/kg/min	SPECT-MIBI	72% (n=142	76% (n=142	66% (n=68)	74% (n=68)	83% (n=75)	67% (n=75)
Marwick, Circulation 1993	>50%	Ad 0.18mg/kg/min	SPECT-MIBI	58% (n=59)	86% (n=59)	52% (n=31)	81% (n=31)	87% (n=38)	71% (n=38)
Amanullah, Am J Cardiol 1993	>50%	AdE 0.18mg/kg/mi	SPECT-MIBI	74% (n=34)	94% (n=34)	-	-	100% (n=6)	100% (n=6)
Hoffmann, Am J Cardiol 1993	>70%	DbE 40mcg/kg/mi	SPECT-MIBI	79% (n=48)	89% (n=42)	78% (n=27)	84% (n=25)	81% (n=16)	71% (n=13)
Takeuchi, J Am Soc Echo 1993	>50%	DbE 30mcg/kg/mi	SPECT-Tl	85% (n=74)	89% (n=74)	73% (n=37)	78% (n=37)	93% (n=46)	85% (n=46)
Gunalp, J Nucl Med 1993	>50%	DbE 30mcg/kg/mi	SPECT-MIBI	83% (n=18)	94% (n=18)	-	-	88% (n=9)	88% (n=9)

AD = adenosine, CAD = coronary artery disease, Dipy = dipyridamole, Echo = ex- ercise echocardiogram, MI = myocardial infarction, ref = reference number, SVD = single vessel disease, Tl = thallium, WMA = wall motion abnormality.

Generally, the sensitivity of perfusion scintigraphy is a few percentage points greater than that of stress echocardiography. Most of these discrepancies are in patients with single vessel disease, in which case the extent of true ischemia, as opposed to flow maldistribution, may be relatively small [26]. Similarly, it might be expected that patients treated with antianginal therapy would be more likely to have discrepant findings, because the development of ischemia is inhibited by the drugs, while flow disturbances are unchanged [10,27]. The results are similarly comparable with regard to specificity, though there is a trend to somewhat higher specificity in favor of stress echocardiography, particularly in patients with left ventricular hypertrophy and left bundle branch block [25].

Three differences which are not apparent from analysis of sensitivity and specificity alone are the identification of ischemia in the setting of previous infarction, the recognition of multivessel disease and cost considerations. In patients with a previous myocardial infarction, hypokinesis may be present at rest, and it may be difficult to appreciate subtle worsening in the severity of hypokinesis following stress, a deterioration of which may indicate the presence of ischemia. When the correlation between ischemia by thallium and stress echocardiography has been examined in groups with and without resting wall motion abnormalities, the concordance was greater in those with normal resting function [28]. In the setting of resting wall motion abnormalities, only 45% of segments were identified as having scar by thallium imaging but 33% were found to be ischemic. Whether this is truly a benefit of perfusion imaging remains to be resolved, although a fascinating recent study has suggested that the detection of ischemia at dipyridamole thallium SPECT following myocardial infarction was not predictive of events over 2 years of follow-up, whereas the detection of ischemia using stress echocardiography was predictive of subsequent events [29]. With regard to the recognition of multivessel disease, the sensitivity of stress echocardiography for recognizing >1 vessel to be involved is >80% in patients with previous myocardial infarction. In those without previous infarction, it is often difficult to identify the involvement of a second territory [9], both because the most abnormal segment is most noticeable, and also because the stress may be limited by the more severe stenosis. This is also a problem for perfusion imaging, although probably less so than for stress echocardiography. Finally, an important benefit in favor of stress echocardiography in the current economic environment is it's cost, which is substantially less than that of perfusion imaging because of less expensive equipment and the absence of expensive disposables, including isotope costs.

In summary, the advantages of echocardiography are the presence of a lower cost for a similar overall level of accuracy, the benefit of fewer false positives (particularly in patients with left ventricular hypertrophy and left bundle branch block), and the nature of the test as being more "patient friendly", because it is shorter and it minimizes multiple testing in patients who also require examination of valves or left ventricular function. Scintigraphy has the advantage of greater sensitivity in the setting of single vessel disease, and more readily detects ischemia in regions of resting wall motion abnormalities. It should be used in patients with suboptimal echo image quality (eg. patients with chronic lung disease and the obese); if a vasodilator stress is to be used because the patient is unable to exercise or tolerate dobutamine, only scintigraphy should be considered.

Prognostic evaluation using stress echocardiography

The use of stress imaging tests for risk stratification in patients with known or suspected coronary disease usually involves three situations. These are the assessment of cardiac risk at the time of noncardiac surgery, the evaluation of risk following myocardial infarction, and the assessment of prognosis in patients with stable chronic coronary disease.

Pre-operative risk stratification

In patients undergoing non cardiac surgery, the risk of a cardiac event in the absence of recent myocardial infarction or congestive heart failure is very small. However, a group which engenders much anxiety regarding coronary risk are the patients with atherosclerotic vascular disease, because of the high prevalence of coronary disease in this group [30]. This high prevalence of coronary disease has two important implications. First, there is risk of cardiac complications at the time of surgery, and second, patients my suffer cardiac events in the years following surgery, which may either reduce the functional capacity that the surgery was designed to improve, or lead to the patient's death. Even in the absence of coronary intervention, major cardiac events (death or myocardial infarction) are relatively uncommon (approximately 5%) in the current anesthetic era [31]. As the pretest probability of an event is low, even using the very best test, the post-test probability will be low even if the test is positive - this probably explains the heterogeneity which has been recorded in the results of myocardial perfusion imaging for risk stratification. Nonetheless, it is important to remember that the justification for preoperative risk stratification in this group is really based on their subsequent outcome. Younis et al. have demonstrated that the presence of ischemia or both scar and ischemia on perfusion imaging confers some major event rate of 30-50% in the 2 years following vascular surgery [32]. While the amount of data available using stress echocardiography for this purpose is less than that obtained to date using perfusion imaging, Table 5 illustrates that the predictive value of a negative test in this situation is comparable to that of perfusion imaging, while the predictive value of a positive test has frequently been in the 30-50% range, as it has been with myocardial perfusion imaging.

Risk stratification after myocardial infarction

Following myocardial infarction, the most important predictor of outcome is the severity of left ventricular dysfunction and the proportion of the ventricle which remains jeopardized. Using conventional imaging approaches, the most efficient strategy for post-infarct risk stratification using cardiac imaging is a combination of echocardiography and perfusion imaging [33]. However, stress echocardiography has the ability to identify both resting dysfunction and ischemia, and may be an efficient technique for

Table 5: Use of pharmacologic stress echocardiography to predict perioperative cardiac events.

Author	Year	n	Stress	PV - positive	PV - negative	Accuracy	Events
Tischler	1991	109	Dipyridamole	7/9 (78%)	99/100 (99%)	106/109 (97%)	MI,AP
Lane	1991	57	Dobutamine	4/19 (21%)	19/19 (100%)	23/38 (61%)	Death,MI,CABG
Lalka	1992	60	Dobutamine	10/30 (33%)	28/30 (93%)	38/60 (63%)	Death,MI,AP,CABG
Eichelberger	1993	75	Dobutamine	5/27 (19%)	48/48 (100%)	53/75 (71%)	MI,AP
Langan	1993	81	Dobutamine	12/25 (48%)	56/56 (100%)	68/81 (84%)	MI,AP,CABG,cancellation
Davila-Roman	1992	91	Db + atropine	17/23 (74%)	68/68 (100%)	85/91 (93%)	MI,AP,CABG
Poldermans	1993	131	Db + atropine	15/35 (43%)	96/96 (100%)	111/131 (85%)	MI,AP,LVF

AP = angina pectoris, CABG = coronary bypass surgery, MI = myocardial infarction,
PV = predictive value

this purpose. A number of studies have confirmed the ability of exercise echocardiography to identify the presence of ischemia and multivessel disease following myocardial infarction [34-36]. Stress echocardiography also has substantial prognostic value in the setting, and the large EPIC study has shown this test to reliably predict patients likely to suffer subsequent cardiac events following myocardial infarction [37]. Indeed, the presence of ischemia at stress echocardiography is more predictive of subsequent events than the results of coronary angiography or standard ECG stress testing.

Risk stratification in stable chronic coronary disease

In patients with stable chronic coronary disease, the results of stress echocardiography have important prognostic implications. Sawada [38] demonstrated that even in the presence of positive ST changes, the finding of a negative stress exercise echocardiogram conferred a benign prognosis. Conversely, we have demonstrated that attempted medical treatment of patients with ischemia at stress echocardiography is attended by a substantial cardiac event rate of about 25% over the subsequent 3 years. Moreover, in a comparable group of patients undergoing myocardial revascularization, this event rate was substantially reduced.

In summary, the results obtained using stress echocardiography before perioperative risk stratification, peri-infarction risk assessment, and the assessment of patients with chronic coronary disease all suggest that the presence of stress induced wall motion abnormalities are predictive of outcome. The relative predictive power of stress echocardiography and perfusion scintigraphy, however, remains to be defined.

Detection of viable myocardium

The rationale for using dobutamine echocardiography for the detection of viable myocardium derives from experimental models of myocardial stunning. In these situations, if a coronary artery is ligated and then reperfused, post-ischemic dysfunction or stunning will be detected as a reduction of wall thickening. If the animal is then exposed to isoproterenol or another sympathomimetic agent, function can be returned to baseline values, and when this agent is removed, the function of stunned tissue deteriorates once more [39]. By careful examination of the low dose response to dobutamine, this analysis may be replicated during pharmacologic stress echocardiography [40,41]. Myocardial viability may be manifest in 2 ways. First, a dysfunctional (hypokinetic or akinetic) segment may improve at low dose and continue to improve a peak dose. This would be expected in the presence of stunning, when there is no ongoing stenosis in the infarct related artery, such as in the post thrombolysis situation. The second expression of this phenomenon would be an improvement at low dose, with subsequent deterioration at peak dose, as the segment becomes ischemic. This is more commonly seen in the setting of chronic coronary disease, under which circumstance regional dysfunction although often attributed to hibernation may be due to recurrent episodes of stunning. Table 6 summarizes the results of several recent studies of stress echocardiography for the prediction of viable myocardium. Interestingly, just as several studies have documented that failure to revascularize viable tissue is associated with a significant event rate at subsequent follow-up, the same appears to be true of viable segments identified using dobutamine echocardiography.

Table 6: Sensitivity and specificity of dobumatine echocardiography for identification of myocardial viabilitiy (segmental analysis).

	Post MI	Patients	Sensitivity	Specificity
Smart, Circulation 1993 @	Early	51	19/22 (86%)	26/29 (90%)
Previtali, Am J Cardiol 1993 @	Early	42	50/68 (79%)	118/168 (70%)
Watada, J Am Coll Cardiol 1994 @	Early	21	55/66 (83%)	43/50 (86%)
Cigarroa, Circulation 1993 *	Late	25	9/11 (82%)	12/14 (86%)
La Canna, J Am Coll Cardiol 1994	Late	33	178/205 (87%)	89/109 (82%)

* Patient-based analysis. @ No revascularization.

The place of dobutamine echocardiography in relation to the scintigraphic approach is for the diagnosis of myocardial viability remains to be defined. Two studies comparing dobutamine echocardiography with positron emission tomography have been published. One confirms a high level of concordance both on a segmental and patient basis between the results of these two techniques [42]. The second study involved a follow-up of a small number of patients [43], among whom the improvement of regional function in response to dobutamine was correlated with subsequent improvement at follow-up in those segments which showed a PET pattern of myocardial stunning (normal perfusion with reduced function). In segments with a PET pattern of myocardial scar, no dobutamine response was detected, and the same wall motion was apparent at follow-up. Interestingly, in patients with myocardial hibernation (a PET metabolism - perfusion mismatch), a response to dobutamine was documented, but improvement was documented at follow-up. It is difficult to draw any conclusion from this small number of patients, a proportion of whom were not revascularized and therefore could not be expected to improve at follow-up. In comparison with thallium imaging, a high level of concordance has been demonstrated with dobutamine echocardiography. Preliminary data suggests that the predictive value of dobutamine echocardiography is comparable to that of thallium using quantitative uptake criteria, and superior to using thallium with visual redistribution criteria.

New developments

The ability to examine both perfusion and function in the heart during exercise and non-exercise stress has been attractive for the evaluation of non-coronary heart disease. New indications for stress echocardiography include the prediction of left ventricular functional response to mitral valve surgery, the analysis of dynamic left ventricular outflow tract obstruction, the assessment of aortic stenosis in the setting of poor left ventricular function, and the evaluation of moderate mitral stenosis in symptomatic patients.

Several exciting new developments are pending in the field of stress echocardiography. First, in respect of non-exercise stress, an automated drug delivery system is in the final stages of approval for clinical use. This system has been used to infuse arbutamine, and rather than stressing the patient using a standardized protocol, the physician controls the target heart rate and the speed at which this heart rate is to be attained, and the computer infuses the drug in proportion to the patients heart rate and blood pressure response. Preliminary results suggest that this approach is comparable in efficacy to existing techniques, and may be of benefit in reducing the personnel requirements and therefore cost of performing non-exercise stress echocardiography. With respect to imaging methodology, tissue Doppler imaging and contrast echocardiography both offer the promise of better resolution of the endocardial border, which may facilitate the performance of quantitative measurements of regional left ventricular function. Moreover, using tissue Doppler imaging, it may be possible to quantitate the speed of contraction of the myocardium, in order to produce a less subjective evaluation of regional left ventricular function. The advent of new contrast agents may enable the analysis of myocardial perfusion using echocardiography [44]. Similarly, using analysis of tissue reflectivity, which changes during ischemia, it may be possible to have another marker of ischemia in addition to the presence of regional wall motion changes during stress [45].

In conclusion, both exercise and non-exercise stress echocardiography are an accurate and cost-effective technique for the identification of coronary disease. In the presence of appropriate expertise, these tests are a feasible alternative to other stress imaging approaches, and new technical developments may further enhance the sophistication of the data obtained from these studies.

References

1. Iliceto S, Rizzon P. Stress echocardiography: ready for routine clinical use? Eur Heart J 1991;12:262-5.
2. Iliceto S, Galiuto L, Marangelli V, Rizzon P. Clinical use of stress echocardiography: factors affecting diagnostic accuracy. Eur Heart J 1994;15:672-80.
3. Crouse LJ, Kramer PH. Exercise echocardiography: coming of age. J Am Coll Cardiol 1994;24:115-6.
4. Armstrong WF. Exercise echocardiography: phase II, convincing the skeptics. Journal of the American College of Cardiology 1992;19:82-3.
5. Armstrong WF. Exercise echocardiography: ready, willing and able. J Am Coll Cardiol 1988;11:1359-61.
6. Broderick T, Sawada S, Armstrong WF, Ryan T, Dillon JC, Bourdillon PDF. Improvement in rest and exercise-induced wall motion abnormalities after coronary angioplasty: an exercise echocardiographic study. J Am Coll Cardiol 1990;15:591-9.
7. Picano E, Lattanzi F, Orlandini A, Marini C, L'Abbate A. Stress echocardiography and the human factor: the importance of being expert. J Am Coll Cardiol 1991;17:666-9.
8. Ginzton LE, Laks MM, Brizendine M, Conant R, Mena I. Noninvasive measurement of the rest and exercise peak systolic pressure/end-systolic volume ratio: a sensitive two-dimensional echocardiographic indicator of left ventricular function. J Am Coll Cardiol 1984;4:509-16.
9. Marwick TH, Nemec JJ, Pashkow FJ, Stewart WJ, Salcedo EE. Accuracy and limitations of exercise echocardiography in a routine clinical setting. J Am Coll Cardiol 1992;19:74-81.
10. Lattanzi F, Picano E, Bolognese L, et al. Inhibition of dipyridamole-induced ischemia by antianginal therapy in humans. Correlation with exercise electrocardiography. Circulation 1991;83:1256-62.

11. Marwick TH. Current status of non-invasive techniques for the diagnosis of myocardial ischemia. Acta Clin Belg 1992;47:1-5.
12. Picano E, Lattanzi F. Dipyridamole echocardiography. A new diagnostic window on coronary artery disease. Circulation 1991;83(5 Suppl):III19-26.
13. Cohen JL, Ottenweller JE, George AK, Duvvuri S. Comparison of dobutamine and exercise echocardiography for detecting coronary artery disease. Am J Cardiol 1993;72:1226-31.
14. Hoffmann R, Lethen H, Kleinhans E, Weiss M, Flachskampf FA, Hanrath P. Comparative evaluation of bicycle and dobutamine stress echocardiography with perfusion scintigraphy and bicycle electrocardiogram for identification of coronary artery disease. Am J Cardiol 1993;72:555-9.
15. Previtali M, Lanzarini L, Fetiveau R, Poli A, Ferrario M, Falcone C. Comparison of dobutamine stress echocardiography, dipyridamole stress echocardiography and exercise stress testing for diagnosis of coronary artery disease. Am J Cardiol 1993;72:865-70.
16. Beleslin BD, Ostojic M, Stepanovic J, et al. Stress echocardiography in the detection of myocardial ischemia. Head-to-head comparison of exercise, dobutamine, and dipyridamole tests. Circulation 1994;90:1168-76.
17. Marwick TH, D'Hondt AM, Mairesse GH, Baudhuin T, Wijns W, Detry JM. Comparative ability of dobutamine and exercise stress in inducing myocardial ischaemia in active patients. Br Heart J 1994;72:31-8.
18. Armstrong WF, O'Donnell J, Dillon JC, McHenry PL, Morris SN. Complementary value of two-dimensional exercise echocardiography to routine treadmill exercise testing. Ann Intern Med 1986;105:829-35.
19. Mairesse GH, Marwick TH, Vanoverschelde JL, et al. How accurate is dobutamine stress electrocardiography for detection of coronary artery disease? Comparison with two-dimensional echocardiography and technetium-99m methoxyl isobutyl isonitrile (MIBI) perfusion scintigraphy. J Am Coll Cardiol 1994;24:920-7.
20. Sketch MH, Mohiuddin SM, Lynch JD, et al. Significant sex differences in the correlation of electrocardiographic exercise testing and coronary arteriograms. Am J Cardiol 1975;36:169-73.
21. Williams MJ, Marwick TH, O'Gorman D, Foale RA. Comparison of exercise echocardiography with an exercise score to diagnose coronary artery disease in women. Am J Cardiol 1994;74:435-8.
22. Sawada SG, Ryan T, Fineberg NS, et al. Exercise echocardiographic detection of coronary artery disease in women. J Am Coll Cardiol 1989;14:1440-7.
23. Marwick TH, Anderson T, Williams MJ, et al. Exercise echocardiography is an accurate and cost-efficient technique for the detection of coronary artery disease in women. J Am Coll Cardiol. In press.
24. Van Train KF, Maddahi J, Berman DS, et al. Quantitative analysis of tomographic stress thallium-201 myocardial scintigrams: a multicenter trial. J Nucl Med 1990;31:1168-79.
25. Marwick T, Willemart B, D'Hondt AM, Baudhuin T, Wijns W, Detry JM. Selection of the optimal nonexercise stress for the evaluation of ischemic regional myocardial dysfunction and malperfusion. Comparison of dobutamine and adenosine using echocardiography and 99mTc-MIBI single photon emission computed tomography. Circulation 1993;87:345-54.
26. Pozzoli MM, Fioretti PM, Salustri A, Reijs AEM, Roelandt JRTC. Exercise echocardiography and technecium 99m MIBI single photon emission computed tomography in the detection of coronary artery disease. Am J Cardiol 1991;67:350-5.

27. Leppo J, Boucher CA, Okada RD, Newell JB, Strauss HW, Pohost GM. Serial thallium-201 myocardial imaging after dipyridamole infusion: diagnostic utility in detection of coronary stenoses and relation to regional wall motion. Circulation 1982;66:649-57.
28. Quinones MA, Verani MS, Haichin RM, Mahmarian JJ, Suarez J, Zoghbi WA. Exercise echocardiography versus 201Tl single-photon emission computed tomography in evaluation of coronary artery disease. Analysis of 292 patients. Circulation 1992;85:1026-31.
29. van Daele ME, McNeill AJ, Fioretti PM, et al. Prognostic value of dipyridamole sestamibi single-photon emission computed tomography and dipyridamole stress echocardiography for new cardiac events after an uncomplicated myocardial infarction. J Am Soc Echocardiogr 1994;7:370-80.
30. Hertzer NR, Beven EG, Young JR, et al. Coronary artery disease in peripheral vascular patients. A classification of 1000 coronary angiograms and results of surgical management. Ann Surg 1984;199:-223-33.
31. Mangano DT, London MJ, Tubau JF, et al. Dipyridamole thallium-201 scintigraphy as a preoperative screening test: a reexamination of its predictive capacity. Circulation 1991;84:493-502.
32. Younis LT, Aguirre F, Byers S, et al. Perioperative and long-term prognostic value of intravenous dipyridamole thallium scintigraphy in patients with peripheral vascular disease. Am Heart J 1990;119:1287-92.
33. Candell-Riera J, Permanyer-Miralda G, Castell J, et al. Uncomplicated first myocardial infarction: strategy for comprehensive prognostic studies. J Am Coll Cardiol 1991;18:1207-19.
34. Armstrong W, O'Donnell W, Ryan T, Feigenbaum H. Effect of prior myocardial infarction and extent and location of coronary disease on accuracy of exercise echocardiography. J Am Coll Cardiol 1987;10:531-8.
35. Jaarsma W, Visser CA, Kupper AJ, Res JC, van Eenige MJ, Roos JP. Usefulness of two-dimensional exercise echocardiography shortly after myocardial infarction. Am J Cardiol 1986;57:86-90.
36. Applegate RJ, Dell'Italia LJ, Crawford MH. Usefulness of two-dimensional echocardiography during low-level exercise testing early after uncomplicated acute myocardial infarction. Am J Cardiol 1987;60:10-4.
37. Picano E, Landi P, Bolognese L, et al. Prognostic value of dipyridamole echocardiography early after uncomplicated myocardial infarction: a large-scale, multicenter trial. The EPIC Study Group. Am J Med 1993;95:608-18.
38. Sawada SG, Ryan T, Conley MJ, Corya BC, Feigenbaum H, Armstrong WF. Prognostic value of a normal exercise echocardiogram. Am Heart J 1990;120:49-55.
39. Ellis SG, Wynne J, Braunwald E, Henschke CI, Sandor T, Kloner RA. Response of reperfusion-salvaged, stunned myocardium to inotropic stimulation. Am Heart J 1984;107:13-9.
40. Smart SC, Sawada S, Ryan T, et al. Low-dose dobutamine echocardiography detects reversible dysfunction after thrombolytic therapy of acute myocardial infarction. Circulation 1993;88:405-15.
41. Picano E, Marzullo P, Gigli G, Reisenhofer B, Parodi O, Distante A. Identification of viable myocardium by dipyridamole-induced improvement in regional left ventricular function assessed by echocardiography in myocardial infarction and comparison with thallium scintigraphy at rest. Am J Cardiol 1992;70:703-10.
42. Baer FM, Voth E, Deutsch HJ, Schneider CA, Schicha H, Sechtem U. Assessment of viable myocardium by dobutamine transesophageal echocardiography and comparison with fluorine-18 fluorodeoxyglucose positron emission tomography. J Am Coll Cardiol 1994;24:343-53.

43. Pierard LA, De Landsheere CM, Berthe C, Rigo P, Kulbertus HE. Identification of viable myocardium by echocardiography during dobutamine infusion in patients with myocardial infarction after thrombolytic therapy: comparison with positron emission tomography. J Am Coll Cardiol 1990;15:1021-31.
44. Porter TR, Xie F, Kricsfeld A, Chiou A, Dabestani A. Improved endocardial border resolution during dobutamine stress echocardiography with intravenous sonicated dextrose albumin. J Am Coll Cardiol 1994;23:1440-3.
45. Picano E, Faletra F, Marini C, et al. Increased echodensity of transiently asynergic myocardium in humans: a novel echocardiographic sign of myocardial ischemia. J Am Coll Cardiol 1993;21: 199-207.

Contrast ultrasound for assessment of myocardial perfusion: promise and pitfalls

J.D. Thomas
Department of Cardiology, Cleveland Clinic International Center, U.S.A.

Summary

While the use of echocardiographic contrast is widely accepted for assessment of intracardiac [1] and transpulmonary shunts, assessment of myocardial perfusion by contrast echocardiography is a relatively new, but growing field. The recent development of several contrast agents capable of transpulmonary passage has lead to much anticipation that qualitative (and possibly quantitative) determination of myocardial perfusion with venous injections of echocardiographic contrast may soon be a clinical reality. This paper will review the physical characteristics of several types of ultrasonic contrast, outline their use in determining myocardial perfusion in a binary sense, and discuss the promise and pitfalls for more quantitative assessment of coronary blood flow.

Contrast Agents

In daily clinical practice, it is possible to obtain very good right-sided opacification with hand-agitated saline, ideally mixed with a small amount of blood and air. The blood acts as an emulsifying agent which stabilizes the bubbles and allows better opacification. Such contrast can readily detect the presence of trace amounts of right-to-left blood flow through atrial septal defects and patent foramen ovale. Because hand-generated bubbles tend to exceed 10 μm in diameter, the vast majority of them are trapped by the pulmonary vasculature, with only one or two bubbles surviving to appear in the left heart after 6 or 8 cardiac cycles. Larger amounts of transpulmonary passage may be indicative of pulmonary arteriovenous malformations, as may occur in chronic liver disease. Smaller and higher density bubbles can be obtained by ultrasonic sonification

E. E. van der Wall et al. (eds.), Advances in Imaging Techniques in Ischemic Heart Disease 101–111.

of either Renografin-76, or human serum albumin. Such agents may be readily prepared in the catheterization laboratory or the operating room for injection. Recently, several commercial agents have been developed which hold out the promise of transpulmonary passage of myocardial contrast.

Albumin microspheres

The only transpulmonary contrast agent currently approved for by the United States Food and Drug Administration for human use is Albunex (Mallickrodt Medical, St. Louis, MO). These microspheres are uniformly less than 6 μm in diameter and thus commonly survive transpulmonary passage to opacify the left ventricular cavity. Although not currently approved for myocardial opacification, experimental studies have demonstrated that with sophisticated image processing, this agent can outline coronary perfusion beds. Albumin microspheres have been shown to have microcirculatory kinetics similar to red blood cells [2] making them excellent potential agents for characterizing coronary blood flow.

Polysaccharide agents

An alternative approach for ultrasonic contrast is to trap air in polysaccharide particles. While one such agent (SHU-454, Echovist, Schering AG, Berlin) has long been available for right heart opacification [3] developments in surface stabilization have yielded an agent (SHU-508a, Levovist) capable of transpulmonary passage. This has recently been shown to enhance the Doppler assessment of left-sided blood flow (such as pulmonary venous flow) with hopes that it may yield myocardial opacification [4].

Phase change contrast agents

An entirely different approach to echocardiographic contrast is the use of compounds which "boil" at body temperature and thus change from liquid to gas upon injection into the vasculature. An example of this is the fluorinated hydrocarbon dodecafluoropentane (Echogen, Sonus, Inc., San Diego, CA). In sharp contrast to albumin and polysaccharide microspheres, which travel in parallel with red blood cells and thus produce very transient contrast effect in the myocardium, phase change agents produce very prolonged opacification of the heart muscle. This renders such agents ill-suited for quantification of myocardial blood flow, which utilizes the *transit time* of the contrast effect, as outlined below. However, the relatively intense and lengthy myocardial opacification may make these agents ideal to determine the presence of coronary occlusion in the acute setting of myocardial infarction and attempted thrombolysis.

Encapsulated inert gases

Improved bubble stability may be achieved by encapsulating inert and poorly soluble gases to prevent diffusion and bubble collapse while passing through the pulmonary vasculature. For example, BR1 (Bracco, Milano, Italy) encloses sulfur hexafluoride within liposomes. It appears that these microbubbles traverse the capillary beds with red cells but may show improved survival.

Qualitative assessment of myocardial perfusion

Most efforts to date have considered only **qualitative** assessment of myocardial perfusion, yielding yes/no or present/absent characterizations of regional myocardial blood flow. They do not attempt to **quantify** the blood flow in physiological meaningful terms, such as ml/min/100 g tissue (as is possible with radioactive or color microsphere injection) [5]. Furthermore, because transpulmonary myocardial contrast agents are largely in the developmental stage and yield poor signal-to-noise ratios on echocardiographic imaging, most clinical applications of contrast echocardiography for myocardial perfusion have involved left sided injections, either in the catheterization laboratory or in the operating room. Following are some of the developmental areas for qualitative characterization of perfusion.

Assessment of myocardial risk area in myocardial infarction

When myocardial contrast is injected into the aortic root when a coronary occlusion is present, the potential infarct risk zone is defined by the absence of contrast. Even following thrombolysis or successful PTCA, myocardial contrast may still reveal a perfusion deficit, known as the "no reflow phenomenon" which portends poor recovery of function in that zone [6]. In a study of 39 patients with acute anterior myocardial infarction undergoing successful reperfusion, Ito et al. demonstrated 9 patients with persistent perfusion defects when sonicated ioxaglate was injection into the left coronary artery. These patients demonstrated significantly poorer recovery of regional myocardial function at four weeks than did those who showed good opacification.

Assessment of collateral blood flow

Contrast echocardiography is the optimal modality for demonstrating the presence of functional collaterals into a region supplied by an occluded coronary artery. By comparing the contrast pattern from an injection in the occluded artery versus one in the contralateral artery, it is possible to define the true risk area of potential infarction. It has been shown that in occlusions with widespread collateralization, there is good return of function following angioplasty, indicating viability of the occluded tissue [7]. Contrast echo thus displays the functional significance of collaterals, often much smaller than the 100 μ limit visible by arteriography, which themselves may not be functional for true perfusion.

Assessment of coronary stenosis and angioplasty

In regions supplied by a stenotic coronary artery, resting myocardial blood flow may be normal. Infusion of an arteriolar vasodilator, such as dipyridamole or papaverine, however, may demonstrate a discrepancy in flow between normally perfused regions and significant stenoses. Following successful angioplasty, the discrepancy between hyperemic perfusion should be reduced.

Use of contrast echo in the operating room

Contrast echo agents may be infused along with cardioplegia in order to demonstrate adequate delivery of the cardioplegia solution. It has been shown with this technique that retrograde perfusion better protects regions in the myocardium supplied by severely stenotic coronary arteries. Contrast echo is also useful for determining the success of graft placement. Injecting into the aortic root while still cross-clamped allows assessment of saphenous vein grafts. However, assessment of arterial graft placement requires direct injection into the graft.

Myocardial perfusion by right sided injections

With the development of transpulmonary contrast agents, the possibility of qualitative assessment of myocardial perfusion from right sided injection exists. It was recently demonstrated that reliable myocardial opacification was obtained from right atrial injections of Albunex. Such injections demonstrated the infarct risk area as well as both adequate perfusion and no reflow phenomenon following varying times of coronary occlusion.

Quantitative assessment of myocardial perfusion

The Holy Grail of contrast echocardiography is quantification of regional myocardial perfusion, particularly from a right-sided injection. The approach proposed to accomplish this uses **indicator dilution** theory. As illustrated in Figure 1, if a bolus of contrast were injected into a chamber of volume V with flow through it at rate Q, then the density of the contrast would demonstrate an exponential decay pattern. The mean transit time can be calculated from the observed contrast curve as shown in the figure. Flow rate would then be given by Q = V/TT.

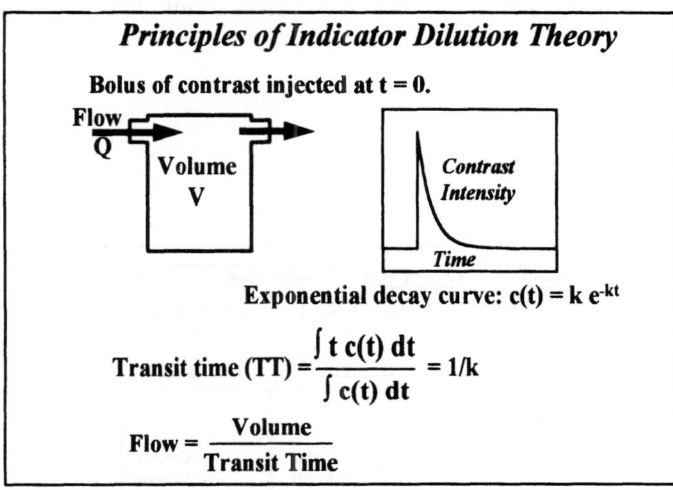

Fig. 1

Requirements of indicator dilution theory

If the schematic in Figure 1 appears too easy to be true, it is [8]. There are stringent requirements on the contrast agent and the imaging and physical systems before indicator dilution theory can be expected to work. Among these are: 1) the contrast agent must be **inert**, passing through the myocardium just like blood; 2) the agent must be **stable**, and not be destroyed as it passes through the body; 3) there must be a **strong**

signal from the myocardium, with a high enough signal-to-noise ratio to quantify the transit time; 4) the **volume of distribution** must be well known to use with the transit time to calculate flow. Unfortunately almost all of the requirements are violated by current approaches to the contrast quantification of myocardial perfusion.

First of all, the situation within the heart is considerably more complex than that shown in Figure 1, since the contrast must traverse many chambers before it reaches the myocardium and therefore displays a broader signal than the spike shown in Figure 1. For example, Figure 2 shows what happens if contrast were injected into one chamber of volume V which then emptied into a second chamber of volume V, then a more complex contrast pattern would occur, broader than the exponential decay curve in the first tank. This curve, termed the **gamma variate function,** is commonly applied in the analysis of indicator dilution curves. Unfortunately, by the time a bolus of contrast reaches the myocardium, it has spread out so significantly that the width of the contrast curve reflects not so much the transit time of the myocardium but rather the broadness of the input signal.

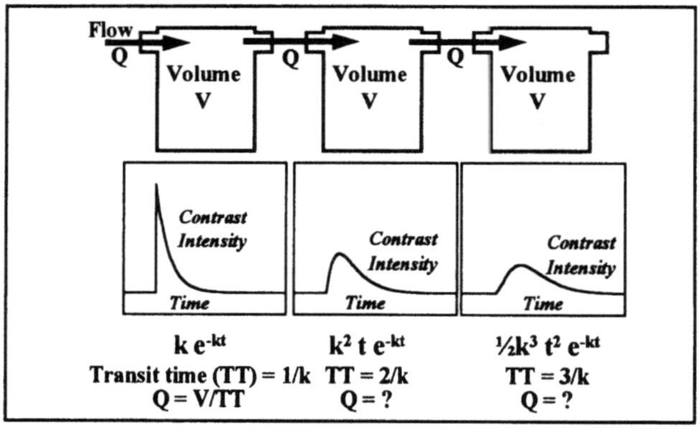

Fig. 2

One possible approach to this signal broadening problem is to analyze the contrast curve just before it enters the myocardium (such as in the aortic root, termed the **input function**) and then within the myocardium (termed the **output function**). Through a method termed deconvolution, it is theoretically possible to extract the **transfer**

function that relates the input curve to the output contrast function observed in the myocardium. Such a technique would hold out the promise of quantification of regional blood flow both at baseline and under hyperemic conditions and in both the endo and epicardium. Unfortunately, deconvolution has such stringent requirements for data quality that it is completely impractical for assessing myocardial perfusion. Among the many significant problems which must be overcome before such a technique can be applied are the following:

1) Indicator dilution theory requires a completely inert substance which is not destroyed as it passes through the blood. Injection of such a substance into a stagnant tank would yield a constant video density. Unfortunately, most commercially available contrast agents display decreased reflectivity at arterial blood pressures, and so video densitometric measurements can only be taken at end-diastole, severely limiting the temporal resolution of the sampling. A recent study utilizing an isolated rabbit heart model demonstrated approximately a 30 point variation in video intensity (in an 8-bit, 256 point image) during the cardiac cycle [9]. This variation was well predicted by a mathematical model of the variation in bubble radius as the gas is compressed at systolic pressures. Because echo reflectivity varies with the *sixth power* of bubble radius, even a minor change in bubble size (4% for a blood pressure of 130 mmHg) will result in a 25% reduction in echogenicity. Furthermore, **there is an irreversible destruction of gas-filled microbubbles** due to the effect of arterial pressure [10]. This leads to a decrease in the total amount of contrast over time, irrespective of the passage of contrast through the myocardium. Figure 3 displays an exaggerated example of the contrast curve which might be observed when gas-filled microbubbles are exposed to cyclic pressure swings in a stagnant chamber. Analysis of the end-diastolic pressure points would yield an exponential decay of video density, implying (by Figure 1) flow through the chamber.

2) The contrast **signal in the myocardium is extremely weak**. Due in part to the random noise present within any myocardial ultrasound signal, the contrast effect barely rises above the noise threshold. Often, the output function recorded is narrower than the input function observed, a physical impossibility unless blood passes through the myocardium in less than zero time.

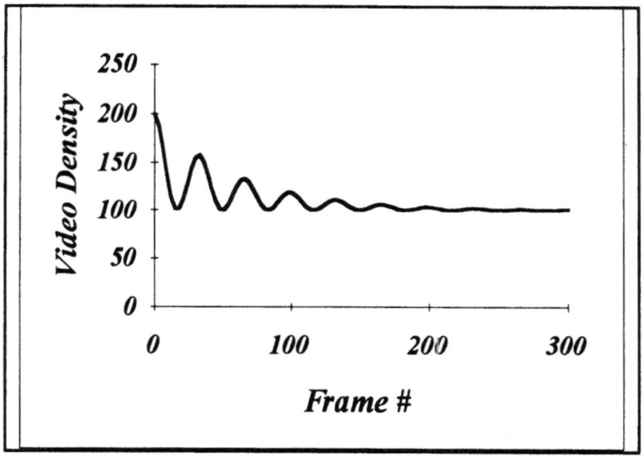

Fig. 3

3) The contrast **injections are not reproducible** at present. Even under ideal circumstances (direct coronary injections using a power injector in an open chest dog model) there was approximately 30% variability between injections for parameters such as transit time and peak opacification [11].

4) The **volume** of distribution must be constant. Unfortunately, under hyperemic conditions, the volume of the myocardium containing blood rises approximately 2-fold, thus making it difficult to quantify flow on the basis of changes in transit time.

5) The myocardial **signal may be significantly shadowed** by echo contrast in a proximal chamber. For instance, right sided injection of contrast passing through the right ventricle will significantly shadow the left ventricle, leading to a decrease in echo intensity, which may not be offset by the increase in myocardial contrast.

Future Directions

Before the quantitative assessment of myocardial perfusion can improve in upcoming years a number of technological improvements must occur:

1) Perfection of **intracardiac ultrasound catheters** with sufficient power to image the entire left ventricle from the right heart. This will permit long-term monitoring of the heart both in the cath lab and in the intensive care unit setting.

2) The development of more **stable contrast agents**, which more completely fulfill the needs of indicator dilution theory.

3) **Improved signal and image processing** with online storage of raw echocardiographic signals and rapid alignment and digital subtraction of pre and post contrast images. Alternate signal acquisition parameters, such as Doppler tissue imaging and 2nd harmonic imaging may yield the kind of signal-to-noise ratio necessary for application of deconvolution to analysis of contrast curves.

If these criteria can be fulfilled, contrast echocardiography may emerge as the optimal technique for assessment of myocardial perfusion in acute and chronic coronary disease.

Contrast Echocardiography for Assessment of Myocardial Perfusion: Key Points

1) Routine clinical use of contrast with hand agitated saline, blood, and air is useful for detection of right to left shunts and transpulmonary shunts.

2) Left sided injections (aortic root or coronary artery) of sonicated renografin or albumin can:
   A) Identify the risk area in acute myocardial infarction.
   B) Identify the presence and function of collaterals around an occluded coronary artery.
   C) Indicate success of reperfusion.
   D) Predict recovery of function following angioplasty of an occluded vessel.
   E) With vasodilator therapy, assess the functional significance of a coronary stenosis as well as the response to angioplasty.

3) In the operating room, myocardial contrast can:
   A) Assess cardioplegia delivery both by antegrade and retrograde technique.
   B) Indicate the most severely compromised zone, to which a bypass graft may be applied initially with further cardioplegia given.
   C) Assess the success of coronary revascularization.

4) Qualitative opacification of the myocardium from right sided injections is in very preliminary stages of development, but appears promising..

5) True quantification of myocardial perfusion, based on indicator dilution theory, appears elusive at present due to:
   A) Instability of the contrast agents.
   B) Low signal-to-noise ratio of the opacified myocardium.
   C) Inter-injection variability in derived parameters.
   D) Variation in myocardial blood volume under hyperemic conditions.
   E) Shadowing of the myocardium by echos in more proximal structures.

References

1. Valdez-Cruz LM, Sahn DJ. Ultrasonic contrast studies for the detection of cardiac shunts. J Am Coll Cardiol 1984;3:978-85.
2. Keller MW, Segal SS, Kaul S, Duling B. The behavior of sonicated albumin microbubbles within the microcirculation: a basis for their use during myocardial contrast echocardiography. Circ Res 1989;65:458-67.
3. Smith MD, Kwan OL, Reiser HJ, DeMaria AN. Superior intensity and reproducibility of SHU-454, a new right heart contrast agent. J Am Coll Cardiol 1984;3:992-8.
4. Von Bibra H, Becher H, Firschke C, Schlief R, Emslander HP, Schomig A. Enhancement of mitral regurgitation and normal left atrial color Doppler flow signals with peripheral intravenous injection of a new saccharide-based contrast agent. J Am Coll Cardiol 1993;22:521-8.
5. Kowallik P, Schulz R, Guth BD, et al. Measurement of regional myocardial blood flow with multiple colored microspheres. Circulation 1991;83:974-82.
6. Ito H, Tomooka T, Sakai N, et al. Lack of myocardial perfusion immediately after successful thrombolysis. A predictor of poor recovery of left ventricular function in anterior myocardial infarction. Circulation 1992;85:1699-705.
7. Sabia PJ, Powers ER, Ragosta M, Sarembock IJ, Burwell LR, Kaul S. An association between collateral blood flow and myocardial viability in patients with recent myocardial infarction. N Engl J Med 1992;327:1825-31.
8. Wiencek JG, Feinstein SB, Walker R, Aronson S. Pitfalls in quantitative contrast echocardiography: the steps to quantitation of perfusion. J Am Soc Echocardiogr 1993;6:395-416.
9. Mor-Avi V, Shroff SG, Robinson KA, et al. Effects of left ventricular pressure on sonicated albumin microbubbles: evaluation using an isolated rabbit heart model. J Am Coll Cardiol 1994;24:1779-85.
10. Vuille C, Nidorf M, Morrissey RL, Newell JB, Weyman AE, Picard MH: Effect of static pressure on the disappearance rate of specific echocardiographic contrast agents. J Am Soc Echocardiogr 1994;7:347-54.
11. Klein AL, Bailey AS, Moura A, et al. Reliability of echocardiographic measurements of myocardial perfusion using commercially produced sonicated serum albumin (Albunex). J Am Coll Cardiol 1993;22:1983-93.

Intravascular ultrasound

Possibilities of image enhancement by signal processing

N. Bom[1,3], W. Li[1,3], A.F.W. van der Steen[1,3], C.L. de Korte[1], E.J. Gussenhoven[1,3], C. von Birgelen[2] and C.T. Lancée[1]

Thoraxcentre, [1]Erasmus University Rotterdam and [2]University Hospital Rotterdam-Dijkzigt, and the [3]Interuniversity Cardiology Institute of the Netherlands

Summary

Cross-sectional frames of intravascular ultrasonic data are the basis of two-dimensional (2D) quantitative information and three-dimensional (3D) reconstruction. A method for semi-automatic 3D image quantification for volumetric study of series of echo slices has been developed. This is based on interactive contour analysis of two perpendicular longitudinal sections obtained from the 3D data as a first step. Intraobserver variations appear to be low.

Backscatter from blood may obscure border lines and severely limit automatic contour procedures and 3D imaging. Image frame averaging methods have been applied with limited success to separate blood from tissue. These methods tend to blur fast moving structures.

New technologies to use the radiofrequency (RF) ultrasonic signal for image improvement are in their infancy, but look promising. These methods include:

1. Extraction of quantitative tissue parameters based on spectral information obtained from the RF signal.
2. Cross-correlation of a time sequence of RF traces. This yields a high value at the wall region against a low value elsewhere. It is shown that with this technique the image can be improved drastically.
3. Another approach is elastography. With intravascular elastography, external sound waves are enforced on the tissue to allow differentiation of wall properties. Calculated simulations are presented.

E. E. van der Wall et al. (eds.), Advances in Imaging Techniques in Ischemic Heart Disease 113–125.

Introduction

Interventional catheter-based therapeutic techniques have become important as they may avoid the necessity of some surgical procedures. Methods to widen a luminal obstruction in an artery include balloon dilatation, tip abrasion, atherectomy and laser ablation. The possibility that restenosis may occur is well documented. Apparently, the therapeutic methods are not yet optimal, or cannot be optimally applied without further knowledge of the obstruction. Intravascular ultrasound (IVUS) has the unique advantage of visualizing vessel wall morphology and pathology beneath the endothelial surface. Many applications have been reported so far [1-6].
The history of intraluminal echography dates back to the very beginning of diagnostic ultrasound. Over the years many fascinating ideas and applications of catheter tip or gastroscopic tube tip mounted transducers have been described. A survey is documented in "Early and recent intraluminal ultrasound devices" [7]. Today catheter tip intravascular echo systems are based on two principles.

Single element mechanical systems

Mechanical rotation of a single ultrasound element permits to scan the vessel wall approximately perpendicular to the long axis of the catheter. Either rotation of the element or of an acoustic reflector in front of a fixed ultrasound element causes the sound beam to rotate, thus building a cross-sectional echo image in real time. An example of an early description of this type of devices dates back to 1966 [8]. All mechanical systems that are presently commercially available are based on rotation of a single element or a mirror in the tip of the catheter. The element or mirror is rotated by use of a long, flexible shaft driven by an external motor. With a long catheter through a tortuous path non-uniform rotation may occur. This could cause image artifacts. The latest development here is substitution of the flex shaft by a micromotor in the catheter tip. The first available micromotor catheter type is built for peripheral arterial applications.

Multi-element electronic systems

A large number of small transducer elements are cylindrically mounted at the circumference of the catheter tip. The signal is processed and multiplexed via ultra-miniature integrated circuits in the tip of the catheter. Signals from each individual transducer element are used for reconstruction of the cross-sectional echo image. This happens in real time [9]. A similar method was suggested as early as 1972 [10]. Although the first commercially available catheters of this type suffered from poor image quality and a large dead zone close to the surface of the catheter tip, more recent catheters have shown a considerable improvement in image quality. The advantage of multi-element electronic echo catheters is the absence of any mechanical drive to rotate the sound beam and the possibility to use a central guide wire.

What can be visualized

Whereas X-ray techniques allow optimal pathfinding for obstruction in coronary arteries by use of contrast fluid, this method does not yield volumetric or morphologic information on the plaque since only the lumen is imaged. IVUS, on the other hand, allows detection of wall pathology, detection of plaque eccentricity and study of the plaque composition. Unfortunately to date, study of plaque composition with IVUS is limited to differentiation between A) "hard" plaques, which are seen as highly echogenic lesions and are likely to be composed of dense fibrous tissue (when shadowing is present, this indicates calcific deposits) and B) "soft" plaques, which are lesions with low echogenicity that may consist of fibrocellular tissue, thrombus or lipid areas.

In addition, since intravascular echography provides tomographic imaging of the arterial wall, quantitative assessment of the free lumen area and plaque area can also be obtained. Usually this is based on manual contour tracing of information in the cross-sectional image. Methods as well as validation of quantitative analysis of intravascular images have been described earlier [10]. The current approach, however, is based on semi-automated analysis of 3D information.

Quantification of three-dimensional information

Quantitative data derived from a single IVUS cross-section have shown to be accurate and reproducible in measurements of vessel cross-sectional dimensions. The slice where the lumen was narrowest has been selected in most studies to date for quantitative evaluation of parameters. However, it is obvious that quantification over the entire narrowed vessel segment is important. Three-dimensional (3D) reconstruction of a sequence of two-dimensional (2D) IVUS images can extend the 2D information to obtain volumetric assessment over an entire vessel segment. The 2D image sequence can be acquired by a catheter pull-back procedure. As an example, over a vessel segment up to 200 IVUS cross-sections were acquired and stored in computer memory. During the image segmentation procedure, a contour detection algorithm based on dynamic programming techniques was applied to both the transversal and longitudinal image data. First, two perpendicular, longitudinal views were generated interactively from the acquired 3D data set. The boundaries of the lumen and plaque were detected from these two longitudinal images, yielding four predefined edge points in the transverse plane, which could be corrected interactively, if necessary. Secondly, using the four predefined points as guidance, the boundaries of lumen and plaque were searched again on the original cross-section. The system accuracy was measured using a 20 mm tubular phantom with an inner diameter varying stepwise from 2 to 5 mm. The result showed a good agreement [13] between true volume and volume measured with the system (true: 212.1 mm^3, measured: 214.6 $\pm$ 2.5 mm^3). To test the reproducibility of the system, five in-vivo intracoronary ultrasound data sets were analyzed two times. Intraobserver variations were low for the measurements of both lumen and plaque volume (mean difference $\pm$ SD: lumen: - 1.4% $\pm$ 3.0%, plaque: 0.2% $\pm$ 1.8%) [14,15]. An example of 3D quantitative IVUS analysis is illustrated in Figure 1.

Given the importance of direct imaging as well as quantitative analysis as described above, a number of limitations exist. On the image quality, for instance, 1) incomplete definition of contours of the lumen and plaque; b) non-coaxial alignment of the ultrasound catheter creating an elliptical distortion and c) non-uniform rotation of the transducer in the mechanical probes. In 3D image reconstruction, problems may be caused by a) inaccurate longitudinal reconstruction if the adjacent cross-sections are not equidistant or b) curvatures of the vessel which induce a spatial distortion of the reconstructed image. Reduction of artifacts and improvement of image quality, in general, are of major importance.

One of the approaches which allow to improve the image quality is to make use of the specific characteristics of backscatter caused by blood.

The ultrasonic backscatter at high frequencies may obscure cross-sectional contours. Ultrasonic backscatter from blood seems to originate from the aggregation properties of red blood cells, as was reported by Van der Heiden et al. [16]. On a series of blood samples experiments were conducted at varying shear rates. The study showed that the shear rate, which is known to influence the state of aggregation [17], has significant influence on the backscatter properties of blood [18,19]. Not only the motion of the blood relative to the vessel wall motion, as it appears on the cross-sectional images in real time, but also the variation with time of rouleaux formation during the cardiac cycle can be used to improve image quality. Obvious first approaches were based on various averaging techniques in the video signal.

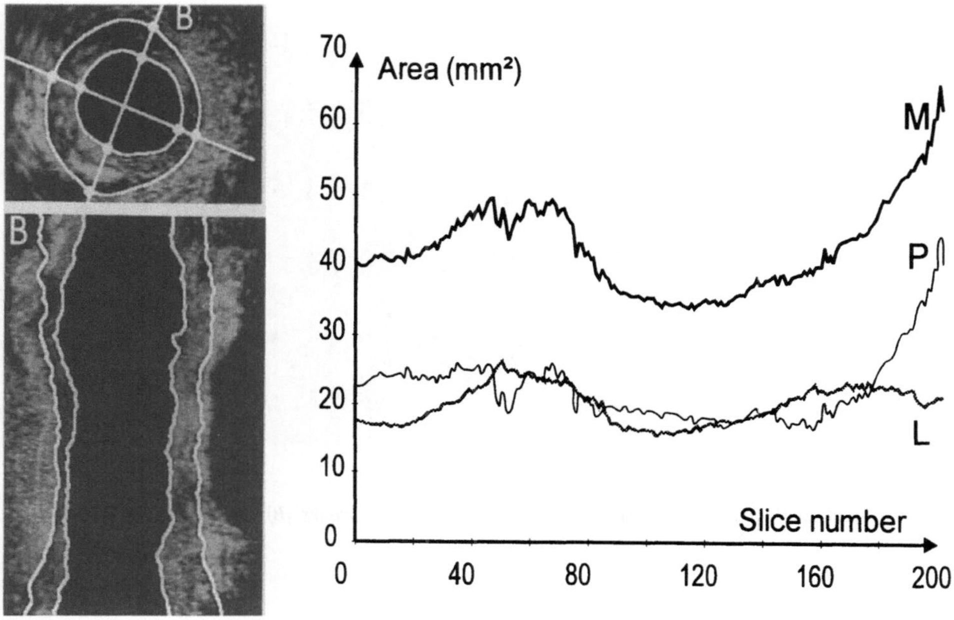

Fig. 1: To the left the first cross-sectional echo image (slice 0; upper panel) is shown as well as the reconstructed longitudinal plane B over all 200 slices representing 4 cm arterial length (lower panel). The area of the media (M), the open lumen (L) and the plaque (P) as a function of slice position are illustrated to the right.

Video signal processing

Using real time IVUS one can see that the backscatter pattern of flowing blood varies over time whereas echoes from arterial tissue present a more static pattern. This phenomenon facilitates differentiation of blood scattering from echoes of the arterial wall on real time IVUS. Because the blood scattering changes with time, averaging a number of consecutive images over time may smoothen out the scattering from blood while preserving the relatively stable structure of the arterial wall, and thus enhancing the luminal interface on a still-frame image. Averaging may be performed using the following formula:

$I_{avg}(x,y) = (I_1(x,y) + I_2(x,y) + \ldots + I_n x,y))/n$

where I represents image intensity, n = the number of consecutive frames at the same cardiac cycle and x,y = image coordinates. An example is illustrated in Figure 2 where the original image (panel A), the averaged image over eight sequential video frames (B), and the image after a saline flush (C) are shown.

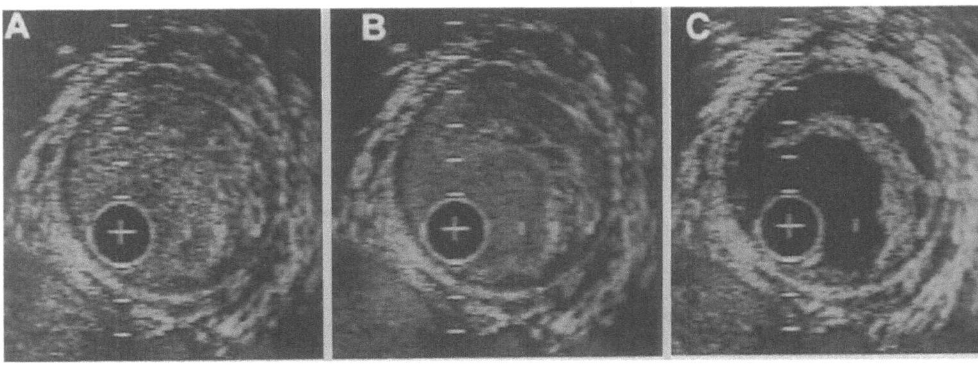

Fig. 2: Original single video frame (A); the averaged image over 8 frames (B); and the saline flush image.

Another approach was described by Pasterkamp et al. [20], whereby sequential subtraction of image intensity was used to improve the image. In order to prevent negative echogenicity the absolute value of the subtraction pixel was calculated.
Representative IVUS images obtained after balloon dilation of the superficial femoral artery are shown in Figure 3: the original image (A), the mean image obtained from 20 consecutive images (B), the mean subtraction image calculated over 20 consecutive images (C), and the saline flush image (D).
One of the major concerns for these sequential video frame averaging algorithms is the possible blurring effect caused by the motion of the wall or the catheter tip. Rapid motion of wall or flaps tend to disappear from the real time image and therefore, in practise, only averaging over a small number of frames is acceptable. Studies on better image processing methods are therefore directed towards the more powerful possibilities using the high frequency RF echo data where faster processing can be applied, thus avoiding a time lag between the video frames.

Examples of radiofrequency signal processing

Quantitative ultrasonic tissue characterization

Integrated backscatter

Integrated backscatter, i.e. the average power of the spectrum of an RF-signal from scattered ultrasound [21,22]. has recently been applied in vitro to various vessels by

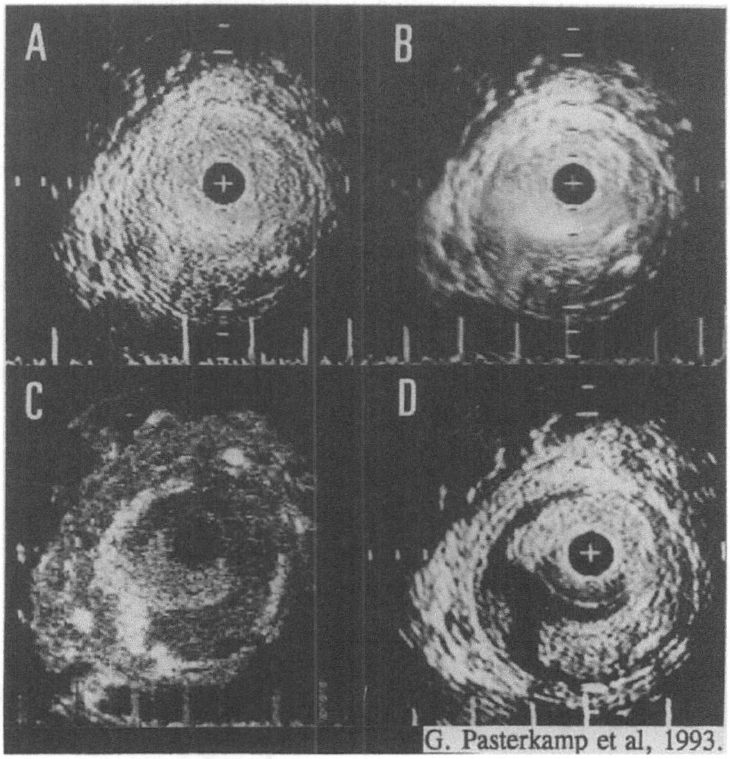

Fig. 3: Representative IVUS image obtained after balloon dilatation of the superficial femoral artery. A: Original image; B: average of 20 consecutive frames; C: Mean subtraction image over 20 consecutive frames, and D: the saline flush image. (With permission from G. Pasterkamp et al. Radiology 1993).

Wickline et al. [23]. Elastic vessels had a higher integrated backscatter than muscular vessels and they found a positive correlation between integrated backscatter and both elastin and collagen. Furthermore, it was shown that it is possible to differentiate in vitro between fatty, fibrous and normal aortic intima. Clinical application of integrated backscatter as a quantitative tissue characterization parameter is complicated by its significant dependence on the angle of incidence [24].

Attenuation-slope mapping

Wilson et al. described preliminary results of attenuation-slope mapping of plaque using intravascular ultrasound [25]. The radiofrequency (RF) data were digitally recorded and used for the calculation of local values of attenuation-slope throughout the tissue using a frequency domain technique. The principle of this method, also described in general literature on ultrasonic tissue identification, is indicated in Figure 4.

It is well known that attenuation increases with frequency. Thus, when the frequency spectra of tissue at a greater depth are analyzed, part of the high frequency components will have disappeared from the spectrum. Obviously this effect is tissue-dependent. As a result the attenuation-slope which is the rate of change of attenuation with frequency can be derived. When the attenuation-slope information is presented as a threshold colour overlay over the conventional image, areas could be identified with differentiation not visible in the original image. These initial results suggested that attenuation-slope mapping might be capable of differentiating between normal vessel wall and fibrous plaque on the one hand and degenerative plaque on the other hand. This may be one of the methods to obtain additional information on wall morphology.

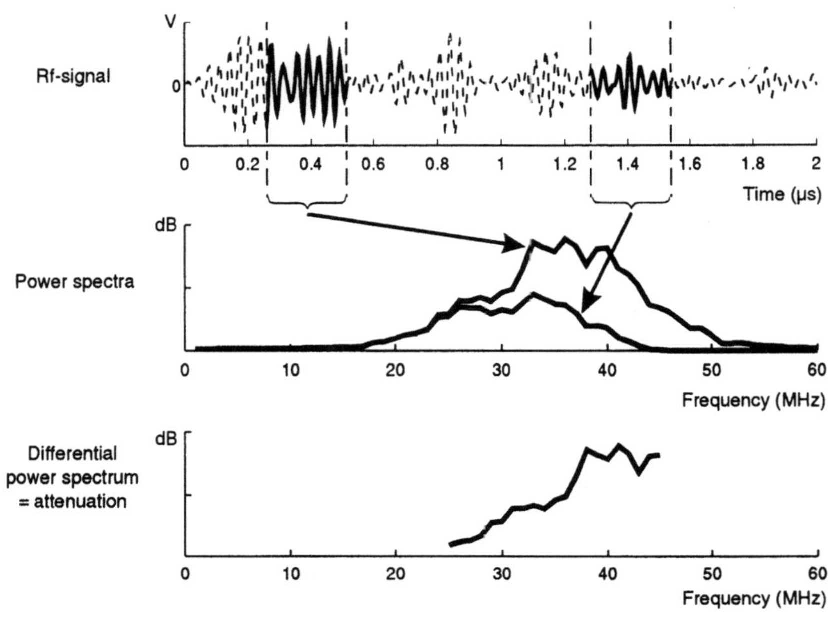

Fig. 4: Schematic illustration of RF spectral analysis as a basis for attenuation imaging.

An RF correlation method

Figure 5 illustrates an RF data processing technique which is able to reduce the visual impact of the blood scattering on the cross-sectional image. Panel A shows a typical normal arterial IVUS cross-section with a fair amount of blood scattering inside the lumen. Along a fixed angular position (indicated by the dashed line), a sequence of RF signals was acquired at 200 μs intervals. The corresponding M-mode data are displayed in Figure 5B with transducer position located at the top. The vessel wall can be appreciated by the difference between the static nature of the wall tissue and the "swirling" blood scattering due to the blood flow. This striking difference gave birth to the idea of using a cross-correlation technique to discriminate between the two. Cross-correlation of a time sequence of RF traces yielded a high value at the wall region against a very low value elsewhere. Using this information as a weighting function, data in panel B were transformed into the image shown in Figure 5C. The blood scattering was completely removed while the vessel dynamics were preserved. After this procedure, the lumen contour could be directly derived from the cross-correlation data for the purpose of quantitative analysis. This technique can be further enhanced by applying a spatial cross-correlation processing on a block of RF data.

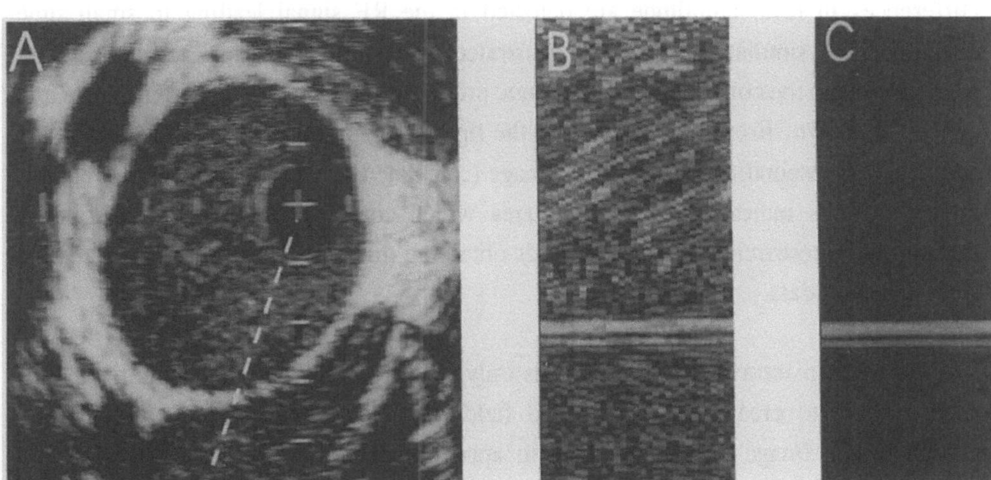

Fig. 5: A: Original cross-sectional scan; B: M-mode data acquired along the dashed line; C: Data processed by cross-correlation techniques.

Feasibility of intravascular elastography

It is well known that mechanical properties of tissue such as elasticity and mechanical impedance differ for different kinds of tissue and change depending on the condition of the tissue. Based on this fact Ophir et al. introduced ultrasonic elastography, a static method to determine the elastic properties of tissue [26]. The essence of this method is based on calculating the correlation between the RF signal from a tissue before and after a small deformation. This reveals information about the local elasticity. In principle this method should be applicable to blood vessels where the deformation would be caused by the systolic blood pressure. It has been applied in vitro to vessels by Foster et al. [27] and Talhami et al. [28], using a pump to pressurize the specimen. Another possible approach is a dynamic one. When an outside sound source is used, local vibration properties will differ depending on tissue properties. Studies are ongoing to calculate the possible feasibility of such an approach. It should lead to detection of local "elasticity" of the vessel wall and the atherosclerotic lesions to generate a complementary image in addition to the normal intravascular ultrasound image. The tissue will be forced to vibrate as a result of a sound wave of, for instance, 10 kHz. The local movement is directly related to elastic properties. The amplitude and the velocity of the local movement represent a mechanical property of the tissue. Differences in local amplitude are detected in the RF signal leading to small time differences. A simulated example is illustrated in Figure 6 where the cross-sectional echo image and the corresponding histologic cross-section from an iliac artery with lipid deposit is shown. From the echo image the lipid deposit area is hardly visible. In the simulated corresponding elastographic image (calculated by C. de Korte), however, this lipid deposit is indicated by the dark area which corresponds well with histology. Elastographic research is directed towards obtaining this type of additional information from the echo data.

Elastography in intravascular imaging is only in its very infancy and huge problems such as how to create the local sound field have yet to be solved. Nevertheless, approaches in image processing seem to appear above the horizon, which allow to differentiate plaques in a more sophisticated way than just in "hard" or "soft" plaques.

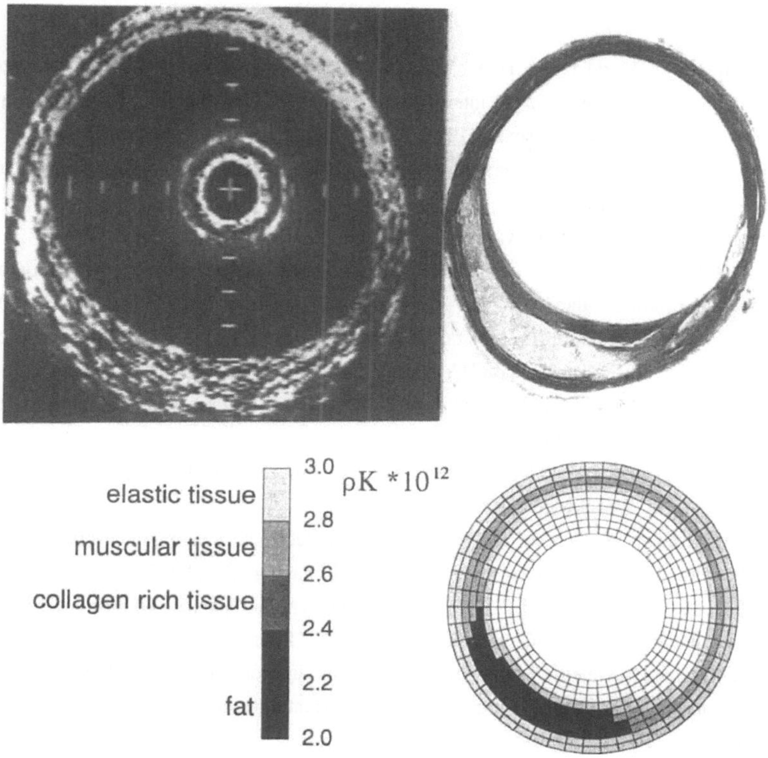

Fig. 6: Echographic (upper panel, left), histologic (upper panel, right) and simulated (lower panel) images of the same vessel segment. The echo image does not show the apparently present fatty area located between 6 and 9 o'clock. Based on practical values for ρ (= density) and K (=compressibility), the simulated image clearly shows the presence of fat.

Conclusions

It is of paramount importance to improve the image quality in intravascular imaging as well as improve the parameter extraction on tissue and plaque morphology. This will further simplify techniques for quantitative analysis of IVUS images. New image processing methods are mostly based on RF signal processing. Some have already shown to be powerful; other approaches, such as the elasticity approach, are yet in their infancy.

References

1. Roelandt JRTC, Di Mario C, de Feyter PJ, van den Brand M, Serruys PW, Bom N. Intravascular ultrasound: instrumentation, image interpretation, promises and pitfalls. In P. Hanrath et al: Cardiovascular Imaging by Ultrasound, 1993, Kluwer Academic Publishers: p. 325-341.
2. Yock PG, Linker DT. Intravascular ultrasound. Looking below the surface of vascular disease. Circulation 1990;81:1715-8.
3. Hodgson JM, editor. Atlas of intravascular ultrasound. New York: Raven Press, 1994.
4. Honye J, Ashit J, Mahon DJ, Tobis JM. Atherosclerotic plaque eccentricity: a comparison of angiography and intravascular ultrasound imaging [abstract]. Circulation 1991; 84: (4 Suppl):II701.
5. Tobis JM, Yock PG, editors. Intravascular ultrasound imaging. New York: Churchill Livingstone, 1992.
6. Gussenhoven EJ, Bom N, Roelandt JRTC, guest editors. Int J Card Imaging 1991;(3-4):145-311.
7. Bom N, ten Hoff H, Lancée CT, Gussenhoven EJ, Bosch JG. Early and recent intraluminal ultrasound devices. Int J Card Imaging 1989;4:79-88.
8. Wells PNT. Developments in Medical Electronics. In: Proceedings of the European Symposium on Medical Electronics. World Medical Electronics, 1966:272-7.
9. Hodgson JM, Graham SP, Savakus AD, et al. Clinical percutaneous imaging of coronary anatomy using an over-the-wire ultrasound catheter system. Int J Card Imaging 1989;4:187-93.
10. Bom N, Lancée CT, van Egmond FC. An ultrasonic intracardiac scanner. Ultrasonics 1972;10:72-6.
11. Li W, Gussenhoven EJ, Bosch JG, Mastik F, Reiber JHC, Bom N. A computer-aided analysis system for the quantitative assessment of intravascular ultrasound images. Comput Cardiol 1990:333-6.
12. Li W, Gussenhoven WJ, Zhong Y, et al. Validation of quantitative analysis of intravascular ultrasound images. Int J Card Imaging 1991b;6:247-53.
13. von Birgelen C, di Mario C, van der Putten N, Li W, Gil R, Prati F, Ligthart J, Camenzind E, Ozaki Y, Serruys PW, Roelandt JRTC. Quantification in three-dimensional intracoronary ultrasound: importance of image acquisition and segmentation. Cardiologie 1995;2:67-72.
14. Li W, von Birgelen C, di Mario C, Boersma E, Gussenhoven EJ, van der Putten N, Bom N. Semi-automatic contour detection for volumetric quantification of intracoronary ultrasound. In: Computers in Cardiology 1994. IEEE Com Soc Press 1994: 277-280.
15. von Birgelen C, di Mario C, Li W, et a. Volumetric quantification in intracoronary ultrasound: validation of a new automatic contour detection method with integrated user interaction [abstract]. Circulation 1994;90 (4 Suppl):I550.
16. van der Heiden MS, de Kroon MGM, Bom N, Borst C. Ultrasonic Backscatter behaviour of human blood in-vitro: manipulated blood samples and shear rate dependence. In de Kroon M.G.M. Acoustic backscatter in arteries, S.L.:S.N., 1993:53-71.
17. Hanss M, Boynard M. Ultrasound backscattering from blood; haematocrit and erythrocyte aggregation dependence. In: Linzer M, editor. Ultrasonic tissue characterization II. Washington: National Bureau of Standards, 1979;525.
18. de Kroon MGM, Slager CJ, Gussenhoven WJ, Serruys PW, Roelandt JRTC, Bom N. Cyclic changes of blood echogenicity in high-frequency ultrasound. Ultrasound Med Biol 1991;17:723-8.
19. Foster FS, Obara H, Bloomfield T, Ryan LK, Lockwood GR. Ultrasound backscatter from blood in the 30 to 70 MHz frequency range. IEEE Ultrasonics Symp Proc 1994;3:1599-602.
20. Pasterkamp G, van der Heiden MS, Post MJ, Ter Haar Romeny BM, Mali WPTM, Borst C. Discrimination of the intravascular lumen and dissections in a single 30-MHz us image: use of 'confounding' blood backscatter to advantage. Radiology 1993;187:871-2.

21. Mottley JG, Glueck RM, Pérez JE, Sobel BE, Miller JG. Regional differences in the cyclic variation of myocardial backscatter that parallel regional differences in contractile performance. J Acoust Soc Am 1984;76:1617-23.
22. Rijsterborgh H, Mastik F, Lancée CT, Verdouw PD, Roelandt JRTC, Bom N. Ultrasound myocardial integrated backscatter signal processing: frequency domain versus time domain. Ultrasound Med Biol 1993;19:211-9.
23. Wickline SA, Miller JG, Rechia D, Sharkey AM, Bridal L, Christy D. Beyond intravascular imaging: quantitative ultrasonic tissue characterization of vascular pathology. IEEE Ultrasonics Symp 1994;3:1589-97.
24. de Kroon MGM, van der Wal LF, Gussenhoven WJ, Bom N. Angle-dependent backscatter from the arterial wall. Ultrasound Med Biol 1993;17:121-6.
25. Wilson LS, Neale ML, Talhami HE, Appleberg M. Preliminary results from attenuation-slope mapping of plaque using intravascular ultrasound. Ultrasound Med Biol 1994;20:529-42.
26. Ophir J, Cespedes I, Ponnekanti H, Yardi Y, Li X. Elastography: a quantitative method for imaging the elasticity of biological tissues. Ultrasonic Imaging 1991;13:111-34.
27. Foster FS, Ryan LK, Lockwood GR. High frequency ultrasound scanning of the arterial wall. In Roelandt JRTC, Gussenhoven EJ, Bom N, editors. Intravascular Ultrasound. Dordrecht: Kluwer Academic Publishers, 1993:91-108.
28. Talhami HE, Wilson LS, Neale ML. Spectral tissue strain: a new technique for imaging tissue strain using intravascular ultrasound. Ultrasound Med Biol 1994;20:759-72.

Clinical aspects of intravascular ultrasound

E.M. Tuzcu
Department of Cardiology, Cleveland Clinic International Center, U.S.A.

Summary

Coronary angiography has been the gold standard for imaging in the diagnostic and interventional catheterization laboratory. This modality depicts coronary arteries as a silhouette of the lumen. The information regarding the vessel wall and its contents are obtained inferentially when they encroach upon the lumen. Recent technological advances have led to the development of miniature intra-coronary ultrasound catheters. This new modality of imaging provides cross-sectional images of the coronary lumen as well as it's wall. Thus, intravascular ultrasound allows accurate measurement of vessel and atherosclerotic plaque dimensions as well as dimensions of other wall components. Moreover, it can characterize the composition and distribution of the atheroma. Experience with intravascular ultrasound imaging has revealed significant limitations of angiographic assessment of the coronary anatomy.

Equipment and technique

Currently available intracoronary ultrasonography catheters range in size from 2.9 to 3.5 F (0.96-1.17 mm in diameter). Despite this small size, the most recent devices have a high image quality and improved handling properties. The techniques required to perform the examination safely, such as careful handling of guiding catheters, placing guidewires, and advancing the catheter through tortuous vessel segments, are borrowed from interventional cardiology. Standard 8-F percutaneous transluminal coronary angioplasty (PTCA) guiding catheters are used (7-F guiding catheters with an internal diameter of 0.081 inches are feasible with some ultrasonography systems). Most ultrasonography devices have a monorail design with a lumen for a standard, 0.014 inch angioplasty guidewire to allow rapid catheter exchanges. Increased flexibility enhances safety and permits atraumatic examination, even in tortuous vessels. However, despite

E. E. van der Wall et al. (eds.), Advances in Imaging Techniques in Ischemic Heart Disease 127–138.

recent improvements, current catheters have handling characteristics inferior to angioplasty balloons. Guidewire "tracking" is occasionally difficult and may require specialized techniques in some tortuous vessels, distal coronary segments, or segments beyond tight bends. Despite occasional limitations, the cardiologist examines the images in "real-time" as he or she advances the transducer to points of interest along the vessel. Images are recorded on videotape for playback in the catheterization laboratory and for additional analysis off-line.

Although all current intracoronary imaging devices operate at ultrasonographic frequencies from 20 to 30 MHz; there are two different technical approaches to transducer design. A single vendor (Endosonics Corp., Ranchero Cordova, CA) offers a 32 element dynamic electronic array. This device relies on the synthetic aperture principle for image generation. The electronic elements are arranged in a circular fashion around the catheter; precise, sequential timing of groups of elements results in a sweep of the ultrasonographic signal throughout 360 degrees of the vessel arc. A high-speed computer reconstructs each pixel by integrating signals obtained from a variable number of transducer elements. This type of system results in catheters with good flexibility and guidewire tracking; operators can safety place these probes through tortuous vessels and into distal coronary segments. Unfortunately, the currently available multielement device has suboptimal image quality, due to specialized transducer materials that constrain acoustic performance, the limitation of acoustic power due to the small size of individual elements, and the requirement for complex computer images reconstruction (which limits temporal resolution to 10 frames per second). Despite these current limitations, a novel combination multielement imaging device and angioplasty balloon called the Oracle Micro (Endosonics Corp., Pleasanton, CA) is being tested clinically. This device has an imaging transducer mounted proximal to a standard balloon. In the future, such a device may enable ultrasound imaging after sequential balloon inflations, allowing the interventionist to remodel the artery in an iterative fashion. However, the optimal strategy for intravascular ultrasonography guidance of balloon angioplasty is as yet uncertain, and in the United States, Food and Drug Administration (FDA) approval of this device has been delayed.

The second technical approach to catheter design is mechanically rotated devices in which an external motor drive rotates a single transducer (or a mirror) at the catheter tip. As we will discuss in the section on artifacts, the motor drive and the catheter tip must rotate in a precise, one-to-one relationship to avoid image distortion during computer reconstruction. Two manufacturers market FDA-approved mechanical catheters in the U.S., Boston Scientific Corporation (Watertown, MA) and Cardiovascular Imaging Systems (Mountain View, CA). The Boston Scientific device uses an ultrasonographic scanner developed by Hewlett-Packard Corporation (Andover, MA). In Europe, an additional system is marketed by Du-MED Corporation (Rotterdam, The Netherlands). These systems typically operate at approximately 1800 rpm and have maximum diameters from 2.9 to 3.5 F (0.96-1.17 mm). In comparison to the multielement array design, mechanical catheters have better image quality due to their higher acoustic power. The higher frequency range (20-30 MHz) improves spatial resolution and provides excellent detail to depths of 3 to 5 mm. However, the handling characteristics of mechanical catheters are somewhat inferior; although they are small and flexible enough for routine coronary imaging, they require care to negotiate tortuous vessels successfully. Most mechanical systems have a monorail design to facilitate rapid catheter exchanges without the necessity for a long guidewire or a docking apparatus. The adjacent guidewire can "shadow" 10 to 30 degrees of the vessel circumference. Recent designs allow an acoustically transparent sheath to replace the guidewire; the operator then advances and retracts the ultrasound transducer through the sheath to interrogate the target segment; this approach also reduces the device profile.

Limitations of angiography

Limitations of coronary angiography has been known for the past three decades. Comparative angiographic and histologic studies of the necropsy specimens revealed significant differences between the quantitative assessment of the lesion severity by angiography and by histology [1-5]. Under-estimation of the lesion severity originates for various reasons. Angiographic determination of the luminal narrowing is based on a comparative assessment. The luminal diameter at the most severe site of the obstructive lesion is compared with the adjacent normal reference segment; however, coronary atherosclerosis is rarely a discreet phenomenon. In early and mid stages of the atherosclerosis development, it is not uncommon to find coronary arteries that are "normal" by angiography. Remodeling of the artery which leads to enlargement of the vessel in order to accommodate the growing atheroma can preserve the lumen. Histologic studies have shown that atherosclerosis is mostly a diffuse process [4]. Thus, it is difficult to find a truly normal reference segment in order to drive an accurate percent diameter stenosis. In the presence of athersclerotic involvement of the reference segments, the percent diameter stenosis will be less severe than it really is. Atherosclerosis narrows the lumen of the coronary arteries in a heterogeneous and complex morphology. This frequently irregular cross-sectional anatomy is represented as a simplified single plane silhouette on angiography. A contrast agent that enters the irregular lumen creates an illusion of larger than true lumen on cine angiograms. The complex morphological characteristics of the coronary lesions are further accentuated after percutaneous intervention. These shortcomings cannot be corrected by computer assisted quantitative coronary angiography methods.

Intravascular ultrasound provides information that is unavailable from coronary angiography. Ultrasound images show the vessel wall and atherosclerosis directly in a topographic perspective. This allows for accurate measurement of the lumen diameter, lumen area, plaque area, plaque thickness and vessel cross-sectional area. These measurements can be performed at any number of cross-sections along the length of the coronary artery. Multiple cross-sectional images obtained from co-distant sites in a coronary segment are being used to reconstruct the three-dimensional anatomy of the coronary arteries. Direct visualization of the atherosclerotic plaque allows the observer to appreciate the complex atheroma's morphology, irregular lumen shapes that occur naturally or following interventions. Intravascular ultrasound imaging has been demonstrated to be more sensitive than angiography in detection and quantification of the atheroma in the coronary arteries. Nevertheless, these two methods are not competing imaging modalities, but rather complimentary techniques for delineation of the coronary pathology. In addition to the dimensions of the atherosclerotic plaque, the content can also be qualitatively assessed by ultrasound. It has been reported that the plaque composition determined by intravascular ultrasound is predictive of the outcome of percutaneous interventions [6-14].

Morphological assessment by intravascular ultrasound

Ultrasound images are determined by the refractive properties of the tissues. In the middle aged or older adult, three distinct layers are seen in the coronary artery wall. The innermost layer corresponds to the tissue from the lumen to the internal lamina. The next circular, echolucent layer is thought to represent media. The deepest layer of the arterial wall is adventitia, which is strongly echogenic. However, this tri-laminar appearance is not constant [15]. The appearance of these structures is probably affected by the age of the subject, the disease process and the type of arteries that were examined. The three layer appearance is frequently absent in the coronary arteries of young people, because the intima is too thin to be detected by current ultrasound systems. If the arteries of the young people are examined with higher frequency transducers, it is possible to identify a tri-luminar appearance that was not apparent with currently available ultrasound catheters.

Ultrasound imaging reveals a wide spectrum of morphological types of atheroma in patients with coronary artery disease. Early atherosclerosis appears as an eccentric intimal thickening, mostly located at a bifurcation sites [16]. These changes are almost never seen on angiography. The relative location of atherosclerosis in the vessel wall is also easily determined by ultrasonography. Many atheromas are eccentrically-located, leaving one or more quadrants of vessel circumference free of atherosclerosis. On the other hand, atheromas may occupy the entire circumference and only leave a central lumen. These concentric atheromas differ from eccentric plaques in regard to their response to interventional procedures. Traditionally, coronary arteriography has been used to assess the eccentricity versus the concentricity of an atherosclerotic lesion. The advance of ultrasound imaging has shown that angiography is an insensitive tool in determination of circumferential location of atheroma. In our study, eccentricity by angiography did not correlate with ultrasound eccentricity [17].

The ultrasound texture of the atheroma leads to classification of the plaque according to echodensity. *Sonolucent atheromas*, which appear less echogenic than adventitia, appear to have a high lipid content according to histologic studies. These "soft" atheromas include plaques with various degrees of echogenicity. Some plaques include echogenic elements similar to blood, while others show echogenicity slightly less than the adventitia. It is thought that the echogenicity is related to the fibrotic elements in the plaque. *"Hard" atheromas* are those with echogenic elements that appear to be more echodense than the adventitia. Histologic studies have demonstrated that these hard plaques are frequently associated with fibrosis. It has been proposed that patients with long-standing coronary artery disease more frequently show hard plaques. The appearance of some atherosclerotic plaques contain particularly bright echos, more so than the adventitia, with attenuation of the signals behind these bright echos. This phenomenon is called "acoustic shadowing" due to attenuation of the sound transmission beyond these structures of bright echos. These bright echos, with acoustic shadowing, represent *calcification*. These morphological characteristics may be important in the planning of percutaneous interventions. Plaque distribution and morphology may help predict the outcome of percutaneous intervention. Lesions with extensive calcification are very difficult to dilate by balloon angioplasty. When they are dilated, the risk of clinical significant dissections is higher [18]. Patients with concentric lesions respond better to directional atherectomy than eccentric lesions [19]. This is contrary to the traditional information provided by angiographic studies.

Intravascular ultrasound in diagnostic catheterization

Limitations of coronary angiography have been well known for some time:

1) Angiography frequently underestimates atherosclerotic disease in the coronary arteries due to the diffuse nature of the process. The percent diameter of stenosis is calculated by comparing the most severe stenosis site with the "normal" reference segments. However, ultrasound reveals that normal reference segments frequently show atherosclerosis, so that erroneous results may arise from estimation of stenosis severity by comparison with reference segments which are not truly "normal". Furthermore, a segment of coronary artery may be severely diseased with normal angiographic appearance if atherosclerosis involves the entire length of the segment in a uniform manner. This may be observed in left main coronary arteries, which appear normal angiographically, but distinctly abnormal by ultrasound [22,23].

2) Eccentric atherosclerotic plaque, particularly in the early stage of the disease, may be missed by angiography despite careful examination by multiple orthogonal projections [18]. Very short, discreet lesions in coronary arteries may appear as "napkin ring" lesions that are difficult to quantify by angiography. Sometimes these appearances are due to kinking of the artery rather than true obstructions. Intravascular ultrasound provides crucial information in these settings.

3) It may be difficult to open-up the area of interest in cases of overlapping branches and tortuous segments. In these instances, it may be particularly difficult to visualize and quantify the osteal lesions by angiography. Ultrasound has been very helpful in interrogating sites that cannot be fully visualized by angiography.

4) In the coronary arteries, enlargement of the vessel accommodates the growing atheroma by a process of remodeling [20,21]. This prevents narrowing of the lumen until the atherosclerosis reaches an advanced stage, so that angiographically-measured lumen size remains unchanged. Nevertheless, the clinical importance of these atherosclerotic plaques should not be underestimated, because they can rupture and lead to clinically significant unstable ischemic syndromes, including myocardial infarction.

Intravascular ultrasound in interventional cardiology

Intravascular imaging before percutaneous intervention provides complimentary information to angiographic examination. This includes the distribution of atherosclerosis along the vessel wall, the involvement of the reference segments by the diffuse nature of the atherosclerotic process, the textures of the plaque (from soft to calcific), and the extent and location (deep or superficial) of calcium. Our observations suggest that ultrasound images enable us to better triage patients to various interventional modalities.

Careful ultrasound imaging before and after angioplasty reveals that plaque fissuring is an important and common mechanism of balloon angioplasty [13,24,25]. This occurs in more than half of the patients; however, stretching of the vessel wall also contributes to the lumen enlargement following balloon angioplasty as well as plaque compression and redistribution of the atheroma [25,26]. Baseline ultrasound imaging may reveal extensive calcification that will increase the risk of suboptimal dilatation and dissections. Similarly, extensive superficial calcification is a contra-indication for currently available directional atherectomy devices. These findings may lead to a change in interventional strategy. Post-angioplasty imaging show the major mechanisms that led to lumen enlargement in a particular case. Only a moderate correlation between ultrasonic and angiographic post-PTCA dimensions has been found. This discrepancy is frequently due to the inability of angiography to accurately represent the complex and irregular cross-sectional profiles of post-angioplasty arterial segments [25-28]. The complex lumen shape post-angioplasty (which includes cracks, tears and crevasses), will give the appearance of a markedly enlarged lumen at angiography, while the ultrasound shows the true area of the irregular lumen. Moreover, the presence of atherosclerosis in the reference segment leads to further underestimation of residual stenosis by angiography. Several ongoing studies are examining the importance of post-angioplasty morphology as determined by intravascular ultrasound in predicting long-term outcome of balloon angioplasty. If certain morphological characteristics are associated with increased restenosis rate, utilization of intravascular ultrasound following balloon angioplasty will be a very important application of this new technology.

Directional coronary atherectomy enlarges the coronary lumen by removing plaque; however, it is possible to obtain a good angiographic result with minimal tissue removal [28]. Ultrasound offers an opportunity to evaluate the amount of plaque removal and extent of residual atheroma. Intravascular ultrasound imaging before intervention provides important information regarding the suitability of a lesion for directional atherectomy. Patients with concentric lesions are more suitable for this procedure than those with eccentric lesions, according to recent ultrasound studies [19]. Angiographic determination of eccentricity often does not correlate with ultrasound assessment. In fact, angiographic studies have suggested that atherectomy is more effective in cases of eccentric lesions. Baseline ultrasound information also provides critical information regarding the presence and extent of calcification. If atheromas are calcified near their luminal interface, it is difficult to cut and retrieve these plaques by directional atherectomy. Some other ablative modality should be employed as the first approach in these cases. Ultrasound imaging, combined with angiography, helps to properly orient the cutter of the atherectomy device. Using branches and other vessel wall structures as a landmark, the cutter can be oriented towards the large atheromatous plaque rather than the normal or near-normal vessel wall, though this may not be possible in some cases where reliable landmarks are lacking. Repeat ultrasound examinations can be used to assist atherectomy in order to safely remove a maximal amount of plaque. Repeat ultrasound examination will help evaluate the site of residual plaque and proximity of the cuts to the vessel wall. It is possible to remove larger plaque volumes leaving residual stenoses of 55% in contrast to atherectomy without ultrasound, which leaves plaques in the range of 60%-70% [6,7,28,29]. While larger lumens will probably decrease the risk of restenosis, aggressive cutting and retrieval of tissue without guidance may lead to serious complications. Future studies with ultrasound-guided atherectomy will establish if the methodology is a safe way to reduce the restenosis rate.

Calcified lesions are difficult to dilate with balloon angioplasty and almost impossible to enlarge by directional atherectomy. Rotablation has been proposed as the method of choice in these type of lesions [30]. Traditionally, angiography and fluoroscopy has been used to assess the extent and location of calcification in the planning phase of percutaneous intervention. However, several studies have established that fluoroscopy significantly underestimates the presence and extent of calcification that is detected by intravascular ultrasound [31,32]. Intravascular ultrasound imaging enables the interventionist to accurately assess the vessel from the standpoint of calcification regarding both extent and location. Furthermore, vessels that are treated with rotablation are frequently diffusely diseased and the normal reference dimensions that are determined by angiography can be misleading. Limited data regarding ultrasound findings in rotablation suggest that fibrotic and calcified elements are preferentially ablated. Rotablation leaves a residual that is circular and averages 15-20% larger than the largest burr used. Ultrasound examination following rotablation allows the operator to assess the near-lumen size, shape and surface and the need for further intervention with another device or balloon [9,30].

Stents are the first devices that have been shown to reduce restenosis [31,32]. The angiographic appearance of enlarged lumen following stenting does not always correlate with perfect stent deployment. Hence, anticoagulation has been used after coronary stenting, but this may result in substantial hemorrhagic complications. In order to prevent these complications, stents have been deployed without long-term anticoagulation using careful intravascular ultrasound examination to confirm proper stent deployment. During ultrasound imaging following stenting, various points need close attention: 1) all struts should be well opposed to the vessel wall, there should be no space between the struts and the vessel wall; 2) if there is a dissection due to previous balloon dilatation, the stent should cover the entire length of dissection and 3) there should not be a significant difference (> 20%) between the area within the stent compared with the proximal and distal reference sites. If the struts are not well opposed to the vessel wall, the stent should be expanded by inflating the balloon to a higher pressure or by using a large balloon. If there is significant inequality in the lumen areas, further dilatations should by performed with additional balloon inflations. If the dissections are extending the proximal to distal to the stented segment, the risk of sub-acute thrombosis increases. Multiple stenting should be considered under these circumstances. The emerging data indicates that properly deployed stents do not need long-term anti-coagulation. Sub-acute thrombosis rates of < 1% have been reported in patients who were treated with antiplatelet therapy following stent deployment.

Intravascular ultrasound in cardiac transplant recipients

Heart transplantation improves the quality of life and prolongs the expected survival significantly in patients with end-stage heart failure [33,34]. Transplant coronary artery disease is the most important cause of morbidity and mortality after the first year of transplantation [35,36]. Transplant coronary disease becomes clinically manifest with advanced heart failure or sudden death due to lack of symptoms in these patients with denervated hearts. Routine surveillance coronary arteriography is performed to detect atherosclerosis prior to a clinical event; however, the diffuse nature of transplant vasculopathy confounds angiographic diagnosis. Due to its unique orientation and perspective, intravascular ultrasound provides an opportunity for identification of early atherosclerosis, and is being increasingly utilized at the time of annual coronary arteriography in cardiac transplant recipients.

Prior histologic studies have suggested that transplant vasculopathy is a diffuse, concentric intimal hyperplasia involving the entire coronary tree. However, recently published intravascular ultrasound studies reveal that transplant coronary artery disease is a more heterogeneous process with eccentric as well as concentric lesions distributed diffusely, but in some instances, also focally [37-40]. Moreover, intravascular ultrasound studies within one month of transplantation, revealed that more than one-half of the patients had evidence of atherosclerosis [16]. This finding demonstrated that part of the disease that is observed in the recipients is in fact transplanted from the donors. The morphologic characteristics of atherosclerosis (i.e. eccentric, focal plaques) are that they are frequently located a bifurcation sites and are very small compared with natural atherosclerosis. Continuing intravascular ultrasound studies will undoubtedly shed new light on the difficult problem of transplant vasculopathy.

References

1. Arnett EN, Isner JM, Redwood DR, et al. Coronary artery narrowing in coronary heart disease: comparison of cineangiographic and necropsy findings. Ann Intern Med 1979;91:350-6.
2. Grodin CM, Dydra I, Pasternac A, Campeau L, Bourasssa MG, Lesperacnce J. Discrepancies between cineangiographic and post-mortem findings in patients with coronary artery disease and recent myocardial revascularization. Circulation 1974, 49:703-8.
3. Isner JM, Kishel J, Kent KM, Ronan JA Jr, Ross AM, Roberts WC. Accuracy of angiographic determination of left main coronary arterial narrowing. Angiographic-histologic correlative analysis in 28 patients. Circulation 1981;63:1056-64.
4. Roberts WC, Jones AA. Quantitation of coronary arterial narrowing at necropsy in sudden coronary death: analysis of 31 patients and comparison with 25 control subjects. Am J Cardiol 1979;44:39-45.
5. Vlodaver Z, Frech R, van Tassel RA. Correlation of the antemortem coronary angiogram and the postmortem specimen. Circulation 1973;47:162-9.
6. Tenaglia AN, Buller CE, Kisslo KB, Stack RS, Davidson CJ. Mechamisms of balloon angioplasty and directional coronary atherectomy as assessed by intracoronary ultrasound. J Am Coll Cardiol 1992, 20:685-91.
7. Suarez de Lezo J, Romero M, Medina A. Intracoronary ultrasound assessment of directional coronary atherectomy: immediate and follow-up findings. J Am Coll Cardiol 1993;21:298-307.
8. Potkin BN, Keren G, Mintz GS. Arterial responses to balloon coronary angioplasty: an intravascular ultrasound study. J Am Coll Cardiol 1992;20:942-51.
9. Mintz GS, Potkin BN, Keren G. Intravascular ultrasound evaluation of the effect of rotational atherectomy in obstructive atherosclerotic coronary artery disease. Circulation 1992;86:1383-93.
10. Nissen SE, Gurley JC, DeMaria AN. Assessment of vascular disease by intravascular ultrasound. Cardiology 1990;77:398-410.
11. Nissen SE, Grines CL, Gurley JC. Application of a new phased-array ultrasound imaging catheter in the assessment of vascular dimensions. In vivo comparison to cineangiography. Circulation 1990;81: 660-6.
12. Sheikh KH, Harrison JK, Harding MB. Detection of angiographically silent coronary atherosclerosis by intracoronary ultrasonography. Am Heart J 1991;121:1803-7.
13. Tobis JM, Mahon DJ, Moriuchi M, Honey J, McRae M. Intravascular ultrasound imaging following balloon angioplasty. Int J Cardi Imaging 1991;6:191-205.
14. Porter TR, Sears T, Xie F. Intravascular ultrasound study of angiographically mildly diseased coronary arteries. J Am Coll Cardiol 1993, 22:1858-65.
15. Fitzgerald PJ, St Goar FG, Connolly AJ. Intravascular ultrasound imaging of coronary arteries. Is three layers the norm? Circulation 1992;86:154-8.
16. Tuzcu EM, Hobbs RE, Rincon G. Occult and frequent transmission of atherosclerotic coronary disease with cardiac transplantation. Insights from intravascular ultrasound. Circulation 1995;91:1706-13.
17. Mintz GS, Pichard AD, Kovach JA. Impact of preintervention intravascular ultrasound imaging on transcatheter treatment strategies in coronary artery disease. Am J Cardiol 1994; 73:423-30.

18. De Franco AC, Nissen SE, Tuzcu EM, et al. Ultrasound plaque morphology predicts major dissections following stand-alone and adjunctive balloon angioplasty [abstract]. Circulation 1994;90 (4 Suppl):I59.
19. De Franco AC, Tuzcu EM, Moliterno DJ, et al. "Directional" coronary atherectomy removes atheroma more effectively from concentric than eccentric lesions: intravascular ultrasound predictors of lesional success [abstract]. J Am Coll Cardiol 1995;25 (special issue):137a.
20. Glagov S, Weisenberg E, Zarins C, Stankunavicius R, Kolletis GJ. Compensatory enlargement of human coronary artereis. N Engl J Med 1987, 316:1371-75.
21. Hermiller JB, Tenaglia AN, Kisslo KB, et al. In vivo validation of compensatory enlargement of atherosclerotic coronary arteries. Am J Cardiol 1993;71:665-8.
22. De Franco AC, Tuzcu EM, Eaton G, et al. Detection of unrecognized LMCA disease by intravascular ultrasound in patients undergoing interventions: prevalence and severity [abstract]. Circulation 1993, 88 (Suppl):I411.
23. Elliott JM, Tuzcu EM, De Franco AC, et al. The left main diameter ratio: A specific index of left main coronary artery disease as validated by intravascular ultrasound. In press.
24. Honye J, Mahon DJ, Jain A, et al. Morphological effects of coronary balloon angioplasty in vivo assessed by intravascular ultrasound imaging. Circulation 1992;85:1012-25.
25. Losordo DW, Rosenfield K, Pieczek A, Baker K, Harding M, Isner JM. How does angioplasty work? Serial analysis of human iliac arteries using intravascular ultrasound. Circulation 1992, 86:1845-58.
26. The SH, Gussenhoven EJ, Zhong Y, et al. Effect of balloon angioplasty on femoral artery evaluated with intravascular ultrasound imaging. Circulation 1992, 86:483-93.
27. Werner GS, Sold G, Buchwald A, Kreuzer H, Wiegand V. Intravascular ultrasound imaging of human coronary arteries after percutaneous transluminal angioplasty: morphologic and quantitative assessment. Am Heart J 1991;122:212-20.
28. De Franco AC, Tuzcu EM, Abdelmeguid A, et al.: Intravascular ultrasound assessment of PTCA results: Insights into the mechanisms of balloon angioplasty [abstract]. J Am Coll Cardiol 1993;21 (2 Suppl A):485a.
29. Popma JJ, Mintz GS, Satler LF, et al. Clinical and angiographic outcome after directional coronary atherectomy. A qualitative and quantitative analysis using coronary arteriography and intravascular ultrasound. Am J Cardiol 1993;72:55E-64E.
30. Kovach JA, Mintz GS, Pichard AD, et al. Sequential intravascular ultrasound characterization of the mechanisms of rotational atherectomy and adjunct balloon angioplasty. J Am Coll Cardiol 1993, 22:1024-32.
31. Fischman DL, Leon MB, Baim DS, et al. A randomized comparison of coronary-stent placement and balloon angioplasty in the treatment of coronary artery disease. Stent Restenosis study investigators. N Engl J Med 1994;331:496-501.
32. Serruys PW, de Jaegere P, Kiemeneij F, et al. A comparison of balloon-expandable-stent implantation with balloon angioplasty in patients with coronary artery disease. Benestent Study Group. N Engl J Med 1994;331:489-95.
33. Kriett JM, Kaye MP. The registry of the International Society for Heart and Lung Transplantation: eighth official report-1991. J Heart Lung Transplant 1991;10:491-8.
34. Bourge RC, Naftel DC, Constanzo-Nordin MR, et al. Pretransplantation risk factors for death after heart transplantation: a multi-institutional study. The Transplant Cardiologists Research Database Group. J Heart Lung Transplant 1993;12:549-62.
35. Olivari MT, Homans DC, Wilson, Kubo SH, Ring WS. Coronary artery disease in cardiac transplant patients receiving triple drug immunosuppressive therapy. Circulation 1989;80 (5 p+2):III111-5.

36. Schroeder JS, Hunt SA. Chest pain in heart transplant recipients. N Engl J Med 1991;324:1805-7.
37. Dressler FA, Miller LW. Necropsy versus angiography: how accurate is angiography? J Heart Lung Transplant 1992;11 (3 p+2):S56-9.
38. Pflugfelder PW, Boughner DR, Rudas L, Kostuk WJ. Enhanced detection of cardiac allograft arterial disease with intracoronary ultrasonographic imaging. Am Heart J 1993;125:1583-91.
39. Pinto FJ, St Goar FG, Gao SZ, et al. Immediate and one year safety of intracoronary ultrasonic imaging: Evaluation with serial quantitative angiography. Circulation 1993; 88:1709-14.
40. Tuzcu EM, De Franco AC, Nissen SE, et al. Intravascular ultrasound in cardiac transplant recipients. In press.

Evolution of quantitative coronary arteriography

J.H.C. Reiber*, L.R. Schiemanck*, P.M.J. van der Zwet*, G. Koning*, B. Goedhart*, J.J. Gerbrands, M.J. Schalij*** and A.V.G. Bruschke*****

** Department of Diagnostic Radiology and Nuclear Medicine, ***Department of Cardiology, University Hospital Leiden, **Information Theory Group, Delft University of Technology, the Netherlands*

Summary

In this paper an overview is given of the current state-of-the-art in quantitative coronary arteriography (QCA) and of anticipated future developments. The conventional QCA approaches with automated contour detection techniques based on Minimal Cost contour detection Algorithms (MCA) have been well established and validated. The functional significance of an obstruction can be assessed by measuring the perfusion of the myocardium at different flow conditions, the Myocardial Flow Reserve (MFR). The development of the Gradient Field Transform approach for the quantitation of complex lesions represents a major step forward in QCA. Future developments are directed towards digital-only analyses, standardization of the file formats (DICOM), the incorporation of computer networks and the analyses of the coronary tree for optimizing the image acquisition.

Introduction

Since the first papers on quantitative coronary arteriography (QCA) were published in 1977 and 1978, this field has grown substantially [1,2]. Two major clinical developments which started in the early eighties have stimulated this growth: 1) the enormous innovation and applications in coronary recanalization techniques (PTCA, atherectomy, thrombolysis, stent, laser, etc.); and 2) the increasing interest to study the effects of new drugs directed at the regression or no-growth of existing coronary artery disease, or the delay in the formation of new lesions [3]. This means that until recently these analytical approaches were used predominantly in clinical trials [4,5].

E. E. van der Wall et al. (eds.), Advances in Imaging Techniques in Ischemic Heart Disease 139–152.

Coronary image processing in general has played sofar a minor role in the clinical decision making process. Most interventional cardiologists still rely on eye-ball interpretation of the severity of coronary lesions expressed in percentage diameter stenosis. During such interpretation, the cardiologist also incorporates the temporal information from the image sequences, contrary to the current application of QCA, which is based on single frames. Comparisons between the visual interpretation and QCA have shown that the qualitative interpretation underestimates the severities of minor narrowings (<30% diameter stenosis) and overestimates the more severe narrowings (>70% diameter stenosis). However, Lespérance et al. have elegantly demonstrated that physicians with a large experience in QCA do not show such large systematic errors anymore; they found a maximal overestimation of only 3% for the severe lesions >70% diameter stenosis [6]. In general, the qualitatively assessed percent diameter stenosis agrees better with the percent area stenosis by QCA. In other words, the cardiologists/radiologists apparently take the functional aspects into account in their interpretations.

Over the last few years an increasing interest has been noted in applying QCA before and during coronary interventions. This enables the operator to size the optimal balloon or stent diameter for a particular procedure and to assess the success of the procedure in an objective manner. Such applications are certainly facilitated by the ongoing improvements in computer hard/software (roughly a 100% increase in performance every 2 years) and the optimization of the user interface, so that results become available within seconds, thereby minimally delaying the angiographic procedure. This application is likely to expand as health insurance companies and governments will follow with increasing interest the cost-benefit aspects of intervention procedures.

State-of-the-art in Quantitative Coronary Arteriography

Methodology of QCA

Since 1977 our laboratory has been active in the development, implementation and evaluation of methods for the quantitative analyses of coronary arteriograms [2]. Until approximately 1988, the 35 mm cinefilm was the only practically useful medium for the storage of the coronary arteriograms. In the second half of the eighties digital X-ray systems were introduced for cardiac applications. It became possible to store the images in digital format in real-time on the large Winchester disks of these systems and to retrieve and display selected images and cineruns on the video monitors in the catheterization laboratory. These digital systems have played a major role in the clinical development of intervention cardiology. If such digital facilities would not be available, the complex intervention procedures could not be done without adding significant additional risks to the patient. However, despite all these technical improvements, the 35 mm cinefilm has continued to be the medium of choice in longitudinal multi-center intervention trials, for the following reasons: 1) standard medium facilitating exchange between participating centers and a core laboratory and 2) high spatial resolution, allowing optical zooming for quantitative analysis [7]. For a QCA analytical package to be applicable in a routine clinical environment, it must satisfy the following requirements:

1. minimal user-interaction in the selection and processing of a coronary segment to be analyzed;
2. minimal editing of the automatically determined results. The user should seldom feel the need to edit the intermediary results, such as the detected contours of the arterial segments;
3. a short processing time in the order of 15 seconds or less;
4. high accuracy and precision in the assessment of the morphological data. This to be demonstrated by extensive studies on phantom and on routinely acquired clinical data.

Over the last several years, we have developed and validated two state-of-the-art analytical QCA software packages, which satisfy these requirements:

1. the Automated Coronary Analysis (ACA) software package for the digital Philips[1] DCI and Integris systems, referred to as ACA-DCI;
2. the QCA-package on the cinefilm and digital based Cardiovascular Measurement System (CMS) of MEDIS[2], referred to as QCA-CMS.

Both packages are based on the same basic contour detection and analysis principles, although each package has been optimized for the corresponding image modality, either the 35 mm cinefilm or the direct digitally stored images. The QCA-CMS and ACA-DCI packages are very similar in design and user-interface. We are convinced that simply defining the start and end point of the coronary segment to be analyzed is the best procedure for segment selection. In the next step, an arterial path through the segment of interest is computed automatically [8]. The contour detection procedure is carried out in two iterations: the first one relative to the detected pathline, and the second one relative to the individual left and right vessel contours detected in the first iteration. To correct for the limited resolution of the entire X-ray system, the Minimal Cost contour

---

[1] Philips Medical Systems, Best, the Netherlands
[2] MEDIS Medical Imaging Systems, Nuenen, the Netherlands

detection technique is modified in the second iteration based on an analysis of the point spread function of the imaging chain, which is of particular importance for the accurate measurement of small vessels.

Calibration of the image data is usually performed on a nontapering part of the contrast catheter following a similar edge detection procedure as for the arterial segment; however, in this case, additional information is used in the edge detection process, knowing that this part of the catheter is characterized by parallel boundaries.

From the left- and right-hand contours of the arterial segment a diameter function is determined, on the basis of which the following parameters are automatically calculated: the site of maximal percent diameter stenosis, the obstruction diameter, the corresponding automatically determined reference diameter and the extent of the obstruction. Additionally derived parameters include obstruction symmetry, area of the atherosclerotic plaque and functional information in terms of the radiographic Stenotic Flow Reserve (SFR-) value and transstenotic pressure gradients. The QCA-CMS provides in addition (sub)segment related data, such as the mean and standard deviation of diameter measurements, and projected vessel areas in the proximal, obstructed and distal segments. Of interest is that as of Version 3.0 of the QCA-CMS software, the algorithms for the calculation of the arterial and reference diameter functions have been completely redesigned according to the requirements described in ref. [9]. As a result, the vessel diameter function is now built up by a much larger number of measurement points, while at the same time the vessel size itself is now calculated along more consistent and intuitively correct directions.

An example of a quantitative analysis with the QCA-CMS is presented in Figure 1. In Figure 1a the detected contours along the proximal part of the LAD artery are superimposed in the image. On this first result page, the most relevant quantitative data are presented in the lower panel. The second result page (Fig. 1b) provides an overview of all derived data.

Table 1: Summary of the QCA evaluation results of the ACA-DCI analytical software package.

	Obstruction-diameter		**Reference-diameter**	
	Systematic error (mm)	**Random error (mm)**	**Systematic error (mm)**	**Random error (mm)**
Interobserver variabilities	-0.02	0.11	-0.01	0.13
Intraobserver variabilities	0.03	0.10	0.03	0.13
Short-term variabilities	0.00	0.19	-0.02	0.22
Medium-term variabilities	0.03	0.18	-0.02	0.34

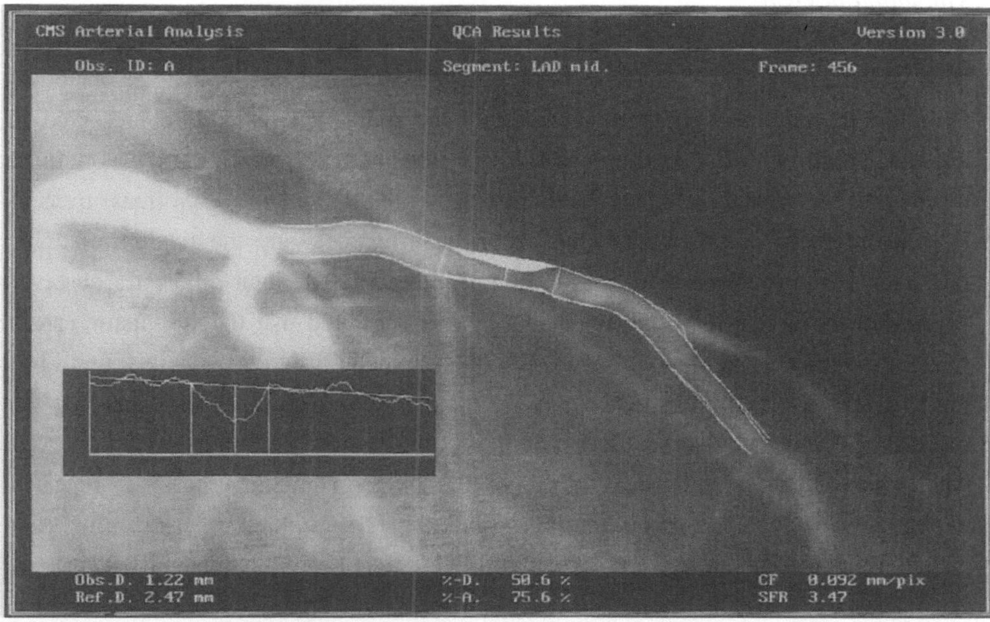

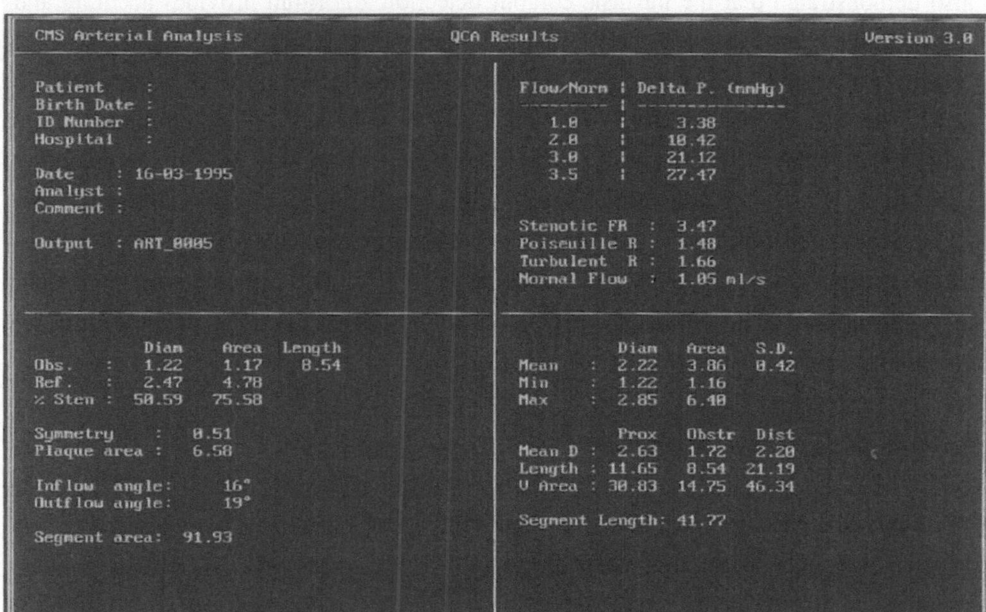

Fig. 1: Example of a QCA analysis on the QCA-CMS. Fig. 1a shows the automatically detected contours, the reconstructed reference contours and the arterial and reference diameter functions. Fig. 1b presents all derived parameters.

Validation of QCA

Both systems (DCI and CMS) have been validated extensively with plexiglas phantoms and clinical materials [7,10]. A summary of the ACA-DCI results are presented in Table 1. In all of the evaluation studies the systematic error or accuracy was defined by the average signed difference between corresponding measurements (measurement 1 - measurement 2, i.e. signed, not absolute difference), and the random error or precision as the standard deviation of these differences. The inter- and intra-observer variability studies on the same set of images demonstrated that the systematic errors were approximately zero, in other words, no systematic differences were found. The random errors for the obstruction diameter were less than 0.11 mm and for the interpolated reference diameter less than 0.13 mm. Larger variabilities were observed when the study was extended to the so-called short-term investigations with repeated angiographic acquisition after 5 minutes and the medium-term investigations with repeated acquisitions at the end of the catheterization procedure under standardized circumstances. These larger variabilities can be explained largely from variations in the calibration procedures on the basis of the contrast catheter. Plexiglass phantom studies also demonstrated that the intrinsic contour detection algorithm provides accurate and reproducible results for vessel diameters of 0.68 mm and larger. With an analysis time of approximately 15 seconds on the DCI-SX, it can be concluded that efficient tools are now available in the catheterization laboratory for the objective and reproducible assessment of the coronary arteries and the changes therein as a result of intervention procedures. Corresponding results with slightly smaller random error values (by 10-15%) were found with the QCA-CMS analytical software package [7]. The performance of the modern CMS workstation (Pentium processor) is such that the computer is not the limiting factor anymore in such applications. Items such as frame selection, documentation of the results, etc. now occupy most of the time.

Myocardial Flow Reserve (MFR)

The analytical packages described above allow the investigator to obtain objective and reproducible data about the morphology of a coronary artery. To obtain a more complete picture about the extent and severity of the disease process, information about the functional significance of coronary obstructions is desired as well. Conversely, in the absence of obstructions in the epicardial coronary arteries, MFR determination provides information about the flow reserve of the microcirculation, which may be helpful in the diagnosis of "small vessel disease"

The approach that we have taken is the one described by Vogel et al. with modifications as suggested by Cusma et al. [11,12]. With this technique the perfusion of the myocardium can be studied at basal and maximal flow conditions. This can be achieved as follows. A bolus of contrast agent is injected during basal flow in the left or right coronary artery, and repeated after the intracoronary administration of papaverine (state of maximal flow). On the basis of a series of subsequent end-diastolic images two functional images are generated for each of the two runs following a mask-mode substraction technique: a contrast-medium-arrival time image (Tarr) and a maximal density image (Dmax) [13] (Fig. 2). From these Tarr and Dmax a relative flow image can be derived. The ratio of these relative maximal and basal flow images is defined as the "Myocardial Flow Reserve (MFR)" image. Finally, MFR-ratio's can be derived for Regions-of-Interest (ROI's) drawn by the user (Fig. 2). This MFR-DCI analytical package is available on the Philips DCI System.
This MFR approach is of particular interest in the following clinical applications [14]:

1. Assessment of the long-term functional effects of interventions in patients with coronary artery disease;
2. Assessment of the immediate functional effects of coronary interventions by calculating hyperemic/hyperemic flow ratios.
3. Evaluation of the efficacy of drugs, in particular their effects on the microcirculation;
4. Assessment of the predictive value of non-invasive tests which have been used to demonstrate the functional severity of coronary artery disease;
5. Clinical decision making in selected patients with coronary artery disease;
6. Diagnostic applications in patients with normal epicardial coronary arteries and signs and/or symptoms of myocardial ischemia. Suspected "small vessel disease" (e.g. "Syndrome X").

Current and future developments of QCA

Quantification of complex lesions

The contour detection algorithm as implemented on the DCI and CMS systems is based on the so-called Minimal Cost Algorithm (MCA), which has been demonstrated to be very fast and robust for images which can significantly vary in quality. This technique has become a basic software tool, which has been applied successfully in other image modalities in our laboratory as well [15,16]. This approach has been demonstrated to work perfectly in QCA as long as the contours are relatively smooth in shape.

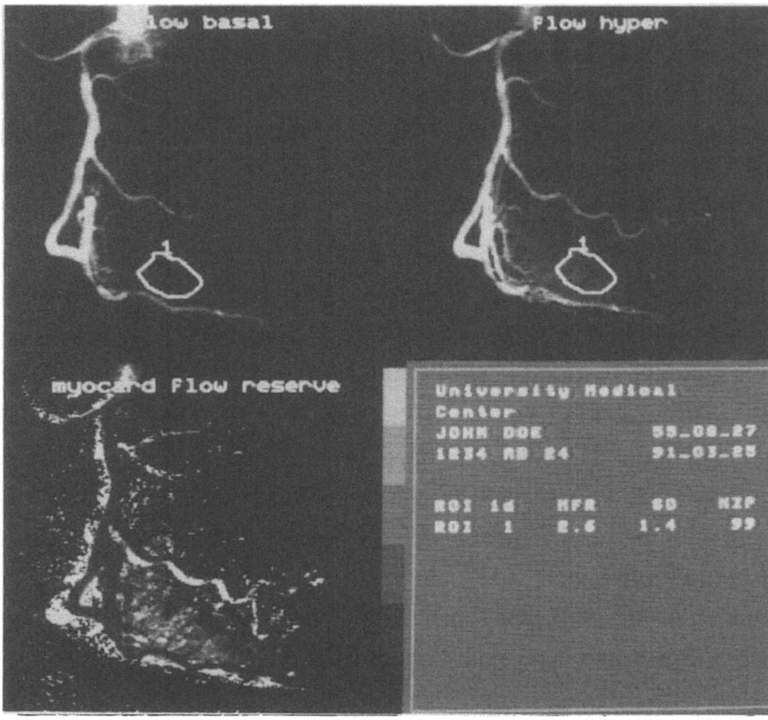

Fig. 2: Example of the result of the MFR-DCI analytical package. The left upper image is the basal flow image, the right upper image the maximal flow image, and the left lower image is the Myocardial Flow Reserve (MFR)-image. The average ± standard derivations of the MFR-values in the manually defined Regions-of-Interest (ROI's) are given in the right lower panel. In this example of a right coronary artery a MFR-value of 2.6 was found.

However, post-coronary intervention obstructions in particular appear to be very complex in shape, for example, when a dissection occurs. Also before intervention, obstructions are found with very sharp corners. Such complex lesions cannot be detected adequately with the MCA-algorithms, for the following reasons: 1) only one contour point can be selected per scanline; 2) the edge strength values are only calculated in one direction perpendicular to the pathline of the arterial segment; and 3) even complex shaped manual corrections are filtered away by the intrinsic limitations of the algorithm.

To be able to adequately analyze such very irregular stenoses, we have developed a novel algorithm, the Gradient Field Transform (GFT), which does not have the disadvantage of the MCA algorithm [17]. The following requirements for this new algorithm were set: 1) the influence of initial models (e.g. the pathline) should be limited as much as possible; 2) all brightness information available in the image must be used; and 3) its speed must be comparable to the MCA. An example of a complex lesion analyzed with the GFT is given in Figure 3.

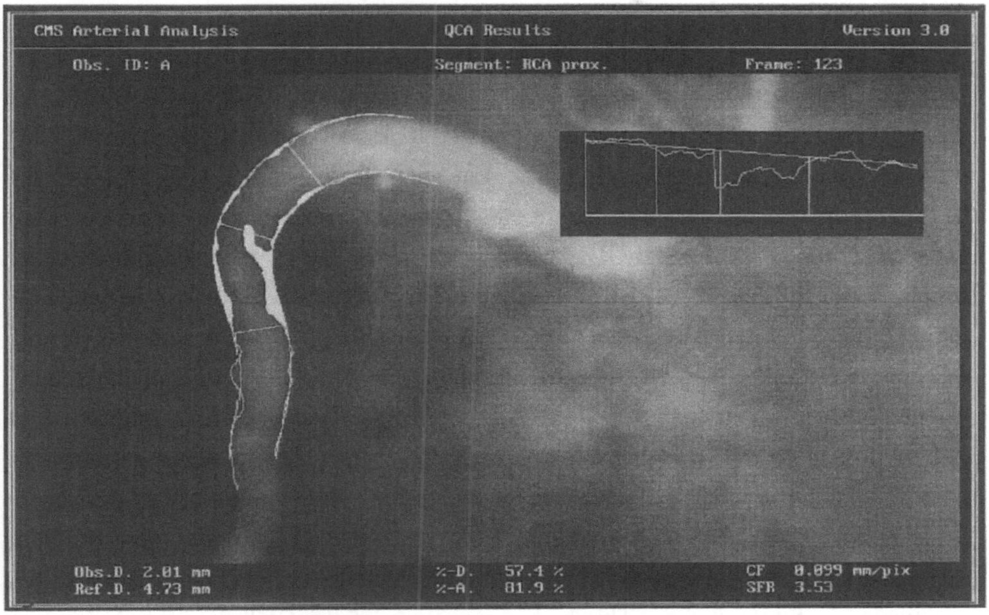

Fig. 3: Illustration of the performance of the Gradient Field Transform algorithm on a complex lesion.

This GFT has been validated extensively on phantom images and on digital coronary arteriograms. In summary, the following results were obtained. In a first study directed towards the assessment of the systematic and random errors of the GFT with a plexiglass phantom with eleven circular tubes (ranging in size from 0.68 - 5.05 mm) which were filled with contrast agent and digitally acquired, a systematic error of -0.004 mm was found and a random error of a 0.114 mm.

In a second evaluation study with twelve copper phantoms with U-shaped obstructions, it was found that even the very severe, very short obstructions (obstruction diameters of 0.5 and 1.0 mm, reference diameter of 5 mm and obstruction length 1 - 2 mm) were quantified very reliably by the GFT algorithm, while these narrowings were severely underestimated by the convential MCA-algorithm.

In a third evaluation study, 25 coronary segments with complex lesions were selected from 19 routinely acquired digital coronary arteriograms. The intra-observer variability in the obstruction diameter was found to be 0.14 mm for the GFT and 0.20 mm for the MCA; for the reference diameter these values were found to be 0.12 and 0.21 mm, respectively.

Based on these results, it can be concluded that the GFT algorithm eliminates the limitations of the convential edge detections algorithm, and therefore it can be useful for the quantification of complex lesions.

The GFT has recently been incorporated into the QCA-CMS software package (Version 3.0) in the following manner and will be implemented in the Philips ACA Version 2 analytical package. The first step in a typical QCA analyses is always carried out following the conventional MCA-approach. Based on the detected contours, the user or the program may decide whether certain parts of the coronary segment are so irregular or complex, that an additional GFT-search is warranted. If so, the user indicates the beginning and the end of the part to be analyzed. Next, the GFT contour detection is carried out and these usually irregular contours replace the local MCA contours. In the usual manner, the user can make further manual corrections. Despite the much higher mathematical and computational complexity of the GFT algorithm, a typical GFT analysis does not take longer than a few seconds. A seemingly disadvantage of the GFT is the fact that the contours, also for smooth parts, are slightly more noisy as compared to the relatively smooth MCA contours. However, these irregularities may provide prognostic information as suggested earlier by Kalbfleisch et al.[18]. This needs to be investigated in future studies. This higher sensitivity of the GFT for irregularities is precisely the reason why we have implemented the current version as an additional iteration on part or the entire MCA-contour. Since complex lesions represent, in general, only a minor percentage of the cases to be quantified, this approach will speed up the analysis of the more regular stenoses.

DICOM and Networking

Until recently, QCA analytical software packages have been developed either for 35 mm cinefilm applications or for digital applications, with the software in the latter case being integrated in the X-ray system console. In the very near future these isolated applications will change significantly for the following reasons:

1. On the X-ray system console of some systems, image analysis and image acquisition cannot be performed simultaneously. In interventional applications this means that the angiographer must wait with the subsequent steps until quantitative data are available, assuming that (s)he wants to base his/her decisions on objective data.

2. There is a great deal of software overhead in the digital X-ray system that slows down the analytical applications.
3. If the QCA is indeed only available on the digital integrated X-ray system and not on dedicated workstations, practice of a busy catheterization laboratory dictates that additional analyses on the X-ray system console are only performed at the end of the day when the patient flow has stopped, or not at all.
4. QCA for clinical research studies should also be possible outside of the catheterization laboratory on remote workstations, connected to a digital Local Area Network (LAN) or a 'sneaker' network.
5. In a few years time the cinefilm will disappear making place for other storage media. To obtain the same accuracy and precision it may be that the matrix sizes have to be increased from 512^2 to 1024^2 pixels. Current developments leading to such scenario's include the definition of the DICOM standard [19], the realization of CD Medical and similar products, etc.

To realize practical solutions at the current state of technology, which will be compatible with the final future solutions, the following steps are anticipated for the QCA-CMS workstation:

1. Recently an on-line QCA-CMS system has been developed which is in use in several major cardiological centers in the USA and Europe. To be able to achieve the necessary performance at present, the input to the on-line CMS is the video signal of the image selected in the cath lab. This image is digitized in the CMS; current analog-to-digital converters are of such high quality that minimal or no information is lost. De QCA-CMS software has been adapted in two ways to make it feasible for on-line use:
   a. inclusion of a digital zoom (bicubic interpolation) for the arterial segment of interest;
   b. optimization of the contour detection algorithms (first and second derivative functions) in MCA and GFT to the characteristics of the digital images.
2. With the DICOM-standard now available and demonstrated at the American College of Cardiology Meeting in March of 1995, the QCA-CMS system can accept DICOM images as well. Further development will lead to the creation of a "digital Tagarno" viewing station, which in its basic configuration will only allow frame selection from the DICOM disks without further quantitation. By adding optional QCA packages, the full QCA-CMS system will be available again.
3. Work is going on to store digitized images either from cinefilm or from the digital medium, and the detected contours and derived indexes if available, in a relational

database on a File Server with a large mass storage device. This will allow a large degree of flexibility to the user, such as:

a. storage of digitized images in the database for later analyses;

b. retrieval of analyzed images plus contours and derived parameters for additional analyses, as is sometimes desirable in regression/progression studies.

c. retrieval of analyzed images plus contours for the calculation of new QCA-parameters which were developed and implemented after the storage of the original data.

d. retrieval of selected images from a baseline study to match the selection of images of a follow-up study, etc.

Coronary Tree Quantification

Based on the desired and expected further automation in the catheterization laboratory and the need to standardize the quality of the acquisitions and the decisions about the extent and degree of the coronary artery disease in the individual patient, it would be of great value if the entire coronary tree could be analyzed automatically or semi-automatically. The computer should indicate the localization (with the proper nomenclature for the segments involved) and degree of coronary obstructions all directly during the actual catheterization procedure. Such an approach will undoubtedly decrease the existing inaccuracies in the visual interpretation, and will lead to a further standardization in the diagnostic procedure and the clinical decision making process.
The first requirement for a successful implementation of such an approach is, of course, an adequate image quality. At this point in time objective criteria to describe the image quality of coronary arteriograms hardly exist. In cooperation with the Information Theory Group (JJ Gerbrands, Ph.D.) of the Faculty of Electrical Engineering, Delft University of Technology, a first step has been made in the automated assessment of image quality criteria [20].
To be able to quantify the entire coronary tree, a technique has been developed in our laboratory to extract the skeleton of the tree, i.e. all the pathlines of the vessels constituting the tree. The only requirement is the manual definition of a starting point, for example in the Main segment at the ostium, and an initial search direction [21]. Next, the arterial contours are detected using the MCA approach. By composing the arterial luminal contours with reconstructed vessel sizes following the principle of the interpolated diameter function, the location and severity of coronary obstructions can be assessed objectively and automatically.

A first start has been made in the automated identification (labelling) of coronary segments from biplane angiographic views using graph matching techniques [22]. Once the three-dimensional description of the coronary tree is available, optimal views for selected coronary segments such that these will be viewed with minimal or no foreshortening, can be calculated. This will be of great practical interest in interventional cardiology. Liénard and Finet have developed and validated such a software tool serving as a positioning guide for the cardiologist; this tool is called COMPAS (Computerized Optimum Method for Profile Angle of Sight) [23].

The preliminary results of our own developments can be summarized as follows. The clinical material consisted of 15 routinely acquired cinearteriograms with a total of 74 vessel segments and 18 obstructions with a severity exceeding 30% diameter stenosis, and 53 digital arteriograms with a total of 236 vessel segments and 69 stenoses. Of the cineframes, which were not magnified optically for this application, 64 (86%) of the vessel segments could be extracted without any user intervention; for the digital images this number was 196 (83%). Repeated (three times) analysis of the arteriograms resulted in an intra-observer variability in the average segment diameters of 0.064 mm for the cineframes, and 0.020 mm for the digital images, and in the minimal obstruction diameter of 0.020 mm and 0.019 mm, respectively. The proximal, mid and distal LAD segments, as well as the septal and diagonal branches, were correctly identified in 86% of the cases.

Although these initial results are promising, further research is necessary to increase the success score of the technique and to be able to apply it on a routine basis.

References

1. Brown BG, Bolson E, Frimer M, Dodge HT. Quantitative coronary arteriography: estimation of dimensions, hemodynamic resistance, and atheroma mass of coronary artery lesions using the arteriogram and digital computation. Circulation 1977; 55:329-37.
2. Reiber JHC, Booman F, Tan HS, et al. A cardiac image analysis system. Objective quantitative processing of angiocardiograms. Comput Cardiol 1978:239-42.
3. Reiber JHC, Serruys PW, editors. Advances in quantitative coronary arteriography. Dordrecht: Kluwer Academic Publishers, 1993.
4. Jukema JW, Bruschke AVG, van Boven AJ, et al. Effects of lipid lowering by pravastatin on progression and regression of coronary artery disease in symptomatic men with normal to moderately elevated serum cholesterol levels. The "Regression Growth Evaluation Statin Study" (REGRESS). Circulation. In press.
5. Bruschke AVG, Jukema JW, van Boven AJ, Bal ET, Reiber JHC, Zwinderman AH. Angiographic endpoints in progression trials. Submitted.

6. Lespérance J, Hudon G, Lemarbre L, Laurier J, Waters D. A comparison of quantitative measurements and visual assessment of coronary stenoses. Circulation 1990; 82 4 Suppl): III-654.
7. Reiber JHC, von Land CD, Koning G, et al. Comparison of accuracy and precision of quantitative coronary arterial analysis between cinefilm and digital systems. In: Reiber JHC, Serruys PW, editors. Progress in quantitative coronary arteriography. Dordrecht: Kluwer Academic Publishers, 1994:67-85.
8. Zwet PMJ van der, Land CD von, Loois G, Gerbrands JJ, Reiber JHC. An on-line system for the quantitative analysis of coronary arterial segments. Comput Cardiol 1990:157-60.
9. Reiber JHC, Koning G, von Land CD, van der Zwet PMJ. Why and how should QCA systems be validated? In: Reiber JHC, Serruys PW, editors. Progress in quantitative coronary arteriography. Dordrecht: Kluwer Academic Publishers, 1994:33-48.
10. Reiber JHC, van der Zwet PMJ, Koning G, et al. Accuracy and precision of quantitative digital coronary arteriography: observer-, short- and medium-term variabilities. Cathet Cardiovasc Diagn 1993; 28:187-98.
11. Vogel R, LeFree M, Bates E, et al. Application of digital techniques to selective coronary arteriography: use of myocardial contrast appearance time to measure coronary flow reserve. Am Heart J 1984; 107:153-64.
12. Cusma JT, Toggart EJ, Folts JD, et al. Digital substraction angiographic imaging of coronary flow reserve. Circulation 1987; 75:461-72.
13. Reiber JHC, Koning G., van der Zwet PMJ, et al. Assessment of myocardial flow reserve with the DCI. MedicaMundi 1993; 38:81-8.
14. Schalij MJ, Geldof MJA, van der Zwet PMJ, et al. On-line assessment of myocardial flow reserve. In: Reiber JHC and Serruys PW, editors. Progress in quantitative coronary arteriography. Dordrecht: Kluwer Academic Publishers, 1994:173-89.
15. Bosch JG, van Burken G, Schukking SS, Wolff R, van de Goor AJ, Reiber JHC. Real-time frame-to-frame automatic contour detection on echocardiograms. Comput Cardiol. In press.
16. van der Geest RJ, Jansen E, Buller VGM, Reiber JHC. Automated detection of left ventricular epi- and endocardial contours in short-axis MR images. Comput Cardiol. In press.
17. van der Zwet PMJ, Reiber JHC. A new approach for the quantification of complex lesion morphology: the gradient field transform; basic principles and validation results. J Am Coll Cardiol 1994; 24:216-24.
18. Kalbfleisch SJ, McGillem MJ, Simon SB, DeBoe SF, Pinto IMF, Mancini GBJ. Automated quantitation of indexes of coronary lesion complexity. Comparison between patients with stable and unstable angina. Circulation 1990; 82:439-47.
19. Anonymous. Cardiac angiography without cine film: erecting a 'Tower of Babel' in the cardiac catheterization laboratory. American College of Cardiology Cardiac Catheterization Committee. J Am Coll Cardiol 1994; 24:834-7.
20. Toussaint CAJ. Development of an objective image quality measure for X-ray angiograms. [M.Sc. Thesis,] Delft University of Technology, 1993 [in Dutch].
21. Dumay ACM. Image reconstruction from biplane angiographic projections. [Dissertation]. Delft: University of Technology, 1992.
22. Dumay ACM, Gerbrands JJ, Reiber JHC. Automated extraction, labelling and analysis of the coronary vasculature from arteriograms. Int J Card Imaging 1994; 10:205-15.
23. Finet G, Lienard J. Optimizing coronary angiographic views. Int J Card Imaging 1995; 11 (Suppl 1):53-54.

Index

MIX
Papier aus verantwortungsvollen Quellen
Paper from responsible sources
FSC® C105338

If you have any concerns about our products,
you can contact us on
ProductSafety@springernature.com

In case Publisher is established outside the EU,
the EU authorized representative is:
Springer Nature Customer Service Center GmbH
Europaplatz 3, 69115 Heidelberg, Germany

Printed by Libri Plureos GmbH
in Hamburg, Germany